Cardiovascular System

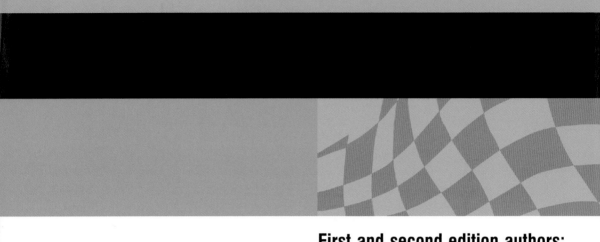

First and second edition authors:

Romeshan Suntheswaran

Toby Fagan

Third edition authors:

Paul Sutton

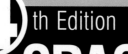

4th Edition

CRASH COURSE

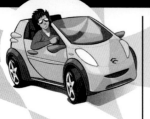

SERIES EDITOR:
Dan Horton-Szar
BSc(Hons) MBBS(Hons) MRCGP
Northgate Medical Practice
Canterbury, Kent, UK

FACULTY ADVISOR:
Professor David Newby
FRCP, FRSE, FESC, FACC, FMedSci
Professor of Cardiology and Consultant Cardiologist
Centre for Cardiovascular Sciences
University of Edinburgh, Royal Infirmary
Edinburgh, UK

Cardiovascular System

Jonathan D W Evans
BMedSci
Medical Student
University of Birmingham

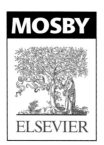

MOSBY

ELSEVIER

Edinburgh London New York Oxford Philadelphia St Louis Sydney Toronto 2012

MOSBY
ELSEVIER

Commissioning Editor: Jeremy Bowes
Development Editor: Helen Leng
Project Manager: Andrew Riley
Designer/Design Direction: Stewart Larking
Illustration Manager: Jennifer Rose

First edition 1998
Second edition 2002
Third edition 2008
Fourth edition 2012
  Reprinted 2013

ISBN 9780723436287

British Library Cataloguing in Publication Data
A catalogue record for this book is available from the British Library

Library of Congress Cataloging in Publication Data
A catalog record for this book is available from the Library of Congress

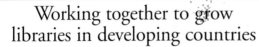
Printed in China

Series editor foreword

The *Crash Course* series first published in 1997 and now, 15 years on, we are still going strong. Medicine never stands still, and the work of keeping this series relevant for today's students is an ongoing process. These fourth editions build on the success of the previous titles and incorporate new and revised material, to keep the series up-to-date with current guidelines for best practice, and recent developments in medical research and pharmacology.

We always listen to feedback from our readers, through focus groups and student reviews of the *Crash Course* titles. For the fourth editions we have completely re-written our self-assessment material to keep up with today's 'single-best answer' and 'extended matching question' formats. The artwork and layout of the titles has also been largely re-worked to make it easier on the eye during long sessions of revision.

Despite fully revising the books with each edition, we hold fast to the principles on which we first developed the series. *Crash Course* will always bring you all the information you need to revise in compact, manageable volumes that integrate basic medical science and clinical practice. The books still maintain the balance between clarity and conciseness, and provide sufficient depth for those aiming at distinction. The authors are medical students and junior doctors who have recent experience of the exams you are now facing, and the accuracy of the material is checked by a team of faculty advisors from across the UK.

I wish you all the best for your future careers!

Dr Dan Horton-Szar

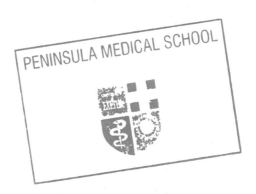

Prefaces

Author

It is my long-held belief that establishing a firm understanding of the principles behind what we learn is far more useful than simply remembering the relevant facts. The cardiovascular system is central to the function of every organ in the human body and a sound understanding of its structure and physiology is paramount. In addition, cardiovascular disease is the leading cause of death in Western society and its importance cannot be overstated.

It is my hope that this book will provide a clear explanation of the basic principles of cardiovascular physiology, and bring these together with an introduction to the common disease processes and the drugs that can be used to treat them. It can serve as a revision aid for the time-pressed student but also provides some extra detail for those students aiming for honours. I do not expect it to replace the more comprehensive texts, but I hope that you find it a valuable addition to your reading that can help clarify points of confusion and save you precious time in the run up to exams.

Jonathan Evans

Birmingham 2012

Faculty advisor

The excellent Crash Course series summarizes the key learning points for the 'information overloaded' undergraduate medical student. The series format enhances learning through concise text, comprehension check boxes, and hints and tips boxes. The key salient points are presented in a user friendly and easy to read manner that enables the rapid assimilation of core knowledge.

The third edition of Crash Course: Cardiovascular System has been updated to provide contemporary emphasis on the cardiovascular system including current concepts of disease and emerging novel therapies. Complementary to the clinically orientated Crash Course: Cardiology, the book highlights all the essential basic knowledge that provides an invaluable foundation for application to clinical practice. The book takes the reader through first principles to inform the basis and presentation of cardiovascular disease, ultimately leading to the investigation and management of common cardiovascular disorders. This logical sequential progression enhances learning and understanding of the cardiovascular system in clinical medicine.

This book is a 'must' for the time pressed student who needs to use their revision time efficiently and effectively in the modern era of systems-based medical education.

David Newby

Edinburgh 2012

Acknowledgements

I would like to thank Professor David Newby for his guidance and support.

I would like to thank all those whose teaching has enthused me about cardiovascular physiology and disease.

I would like to thank Shaan Dudani for his feedback and constructive criticism.

Figure acknowledgements

Fig. 2.3 courtesy of Professor Dame M Turner-Warwick, Dr M Hodson, Professor B Corrin, and Dr I Kerr

Figs 2.30 and 2.31 redrawn with permission from WJ Larsen. Human Embryology, 2nd edition. Churchill Livingstone, 1997

Figs 2.34–2.40 courtesy of T Lissauer and G Clayden. Illustrated Textbook of Paediatrics, 2nd edition. Mosby, 2001

Fig. 2.44 redrawn with permission from Tortora GJ, Grabowski SR Principles of anatomy and physiology, 9th edition. New York: John Wiley & Sons, 2000.

Fig. 2.45A redrawn with permission from PL Williams, ed. Gray's Anatomy, 37th edition. Churchill Livingstone, 1989

Fig. 2.45B redrawn with permission from A Davies, AGH Blakeley and C Kidd. Human Physiology. Churchill Livingstone, 2001

Fig. 2.46 adapted with permission from Burton AC. Physiol Rev. 34: 619, 1954

Fig. 2.50 redrawn with permission from A Stevens and J Lowe. Human Histology, 2nd edition. Mosby, 1997

Fig. 2.53 adapted from Levick R. Introducing Cardiovascular Physiology. Butterworth–Heinemann, 1995. Reproduced by permission of Edward Arnold Ltd

Fig. 3.11 redrawn with permission from O Epstein, D Perkin, D de Bono and J Cookson, eds. Clinical Examination, 2nd edition. Mosby International, 1997

Fig. 3.20 Reproduced with the kind permission of the Resuscitation Council (UK)

Figs 4.8A&B and 9.4 courtesy of Dr A Timmis and Dr S Brecker

Figs 7.7–7.9, 7.13 and 8.6 courtesy of DE Newby and Neil R Grubb. Cardiology, an Illustrated Colour Text, 1st edition. Elsevier, 2005

Figs 7.11 and 7.12 reproduced with permission from A Anand. Crash Course Pathology 3rd edition. Mosby, 2007.

Dedication

For my Mum, Dad and Rebecca.

Contents

Overview of the cardiovascular system

● **Objectives**

You should be able to:
- Describe the functions of the cardiovascular system.
- Explain how the two circulations are organized.
- Understand how the flow and distribution of blood through the two circulations is governed.

WHY DO WE NEED A CARDIOVASCULAR SYSTEM?

The cardiovascular system serves to provide rapid transport of nutrients to the tissues in the body and allow rapid removal of waste products. In smaller, less complex organisms than the human body there is no such system because their needs can be met by simple diffusion. Evolution of the cardiovascular system provided a means of aiding the diffusion process, allowing the development of larger organisms. The cardiovascular system allows nutrients:

- To diffuse into the system at their source (e.g. oxygen from the alveoli).
- To travel long distances quickly.
- To diffuse into tissues where they are needed (e.g. oxygen to working muscle).

This type of process is called convective transport, and is an active process (i.e. it requires energy). This energy is provided by the heart. The functions of the cardiovascular system rely on a medium for transport. This medium is blood, which is made up of cells (mainly red and white blood cells) and plasma (water, proteins, electrolytes, etc.).

FUNCTIONS OF THE CARDIOVASCULAR SYSTEM

The main functions of the cardiovascular system are:

- Rapid transport of nutrients (oxygen, amino acids, glucose, fatty acids, water, etc.).
- Removal of waste products of metabolism (carbon dioxide, urea, creatinine, etc.).
- Hormonal control, by transporting hormones to their target organs and by secreting its own hormones (e.g. atrial natriuretic peptide).
- Temperature regulation, by controlling heat distribution between the body core and the skin.

- Reproduction, by producing erection of the penis and nutrition to the fetus via a complex system of placental blood flow.
- Host defence, transporting immune cells, antigen and other mediators (e.g. antibody).

THE HEART AND CIRCULATION

The heart is a double pump. It consists of two muscular pumps (the left and right ventricles). Each pump has its own reservoir (the left and right atrium). The two pumps each serve a different circulation. In a normal person, every blood cell flows first in one circulation and then moves into the other.

The right ventricle is the pump for the pulmonary circulation. It receives blood from the right atrium, which is then pumped into the lungs through the pulmonary artery. Here it is oxygenated and gives up carbon dioxide; it then returns to the left atrium of the heart via the pulmonary veins and then enters the left ventricle.

The left ventricle is the pump for the systemic circulation. Blood is pumped from the left ventricle to the rest of the body via the aorta. In the tissues of the body, nutrients and waste products are exchanged. Blood (which now carries less oxygen and more carbon dioxide) returns to the right atrium via the superior and inferior vena cavae. The two circulations operate simultaneously and are arranged in series. Unidirectional flow is ensured by the presence of valves in the heart and veins (Fig. 1.1).

The circulatory system is made up of arteries, veins, capillaries, and lymphatic vessels:

- Arteries transport blood from the heart to the body tissues.
- Capillaries are where diffusion of nutrients and waste products takes place.
- Veins return blood from the tissues to the heart. (The hepatic portal vein is an exception. This transports blood from the intestines to the liver.)

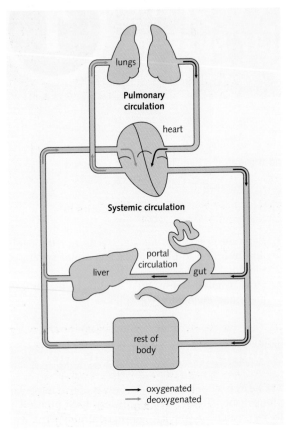

oxygenated
deoxygenated

Fig. 1.1 Systemic and pulmonary circulations. Unidirectional flow is maintained by valves in the heart, pressure difference in the arterial tree and valves in the venous system.

- Lymphatic vessels return to the blood any excess water and nutrients that have diffused out of the capillaries.

HINTS AND TIPS

Arteries carry oxygenated blood and veins carry deoxygenated blood. The two exceptions to this rule are the pulmonary and umbilical vessels (supplying the fetus) where this is reversed.

The amount of blood ejected from one ventricle during 1 minute is called the cardiac output. The cardiac output of each ventricle is equal overall, but there may be occasional beat-by-beat variation. The entire cardiac output of the right ventricle passes through the lungs and into the left side of the heart. The cardiac output of the left ventricle passes into the aorta, and it is distributed to various organs and tissues according to their metabolic requirements or particular functions (e.g. the kidney receives 20% of cardiac output so that its excretory function can be maintained). This distribution can be changed to meet changes in demand (e.g. during exercise, the flow to the skeletal muscle is increased considerably).

Blood is driven along the vessels by pressure. This pressure, which is produced by the ejection of blood from the ventricles, is highest in the aorta (about 120 mmHg above atmospheric pressure) and lowest in the great veins (almost atmospheric). It is this pressure difference that moves blood through the arterial tree, through the capillaries, and into the veins.

ANATOMY

The mediastinum

This is the space between the two pleural cavities. It contains all the structures of the chest except the lungs and pleura. The mediastinum extends from the superior thoracic aperture to the diaphragm and from the sternum to the vertebrae and is divided into superior and inferior parts by the plane passing from the sternal angle to the T4/T5 intervertebral disc. The inferior mediastinum is then further subdivided into anterior, middle and posterior parts (Fig. 2.1). The contents of each part are shown in (Fig. 2.2). The structures in the mediastinum are surrounded by loose connective tissue, nerves, blood and lymph vessels. It can accommodate movement and volume changes.

The heart is in the middle mediastinum, and it has the following relations:

- Superiorly, the great vessels and bronchi.
- Inferiorly, the diaphragm.
- Laterally, the pleurae and lungs.
- Anteriorly, the thymus.
- Posteriorly, the oesophagus.

The structures visible on a normal chest x-ray are shown in Fig. 2.3.

Pericardium

This is the fibroserous sac that surrounds the heart. It consists of two layers, between which there is a small amount of pericardial fluid (see box). The pericardium is fused with the central tendon of the diaphragm at its base, the sternum by the sternopericardial ligament anteriorly and with the tunica adventitia of the great vessels.

> When fluid accumulates within the pericardial sac this is called a pericardial effusion. If it accumulates quickly and begins to affect cardiac function it is called cardiac tamponade. (Both are described in Ch. 8.)

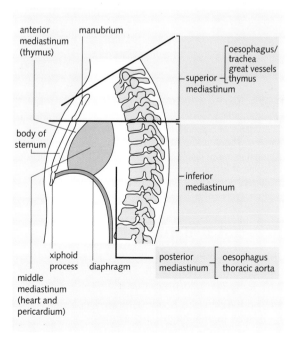

Fig. 2.1 Lateral view of the mediastinum.

Fig.2.2 Contents of the mediastinum	
Superior	Great vessels
	Thymus
	Trachea
	Oesophagus
Anterior	Internal mammary artery
Middle	Heart
	Origins of the great vessels
Posterior	Descending aorta
	Oesophagus
	Sympathetic chain

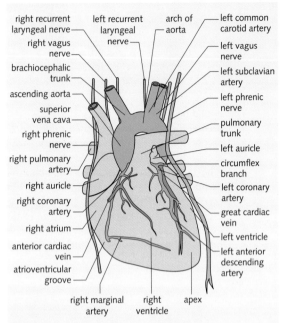

Fig. 2.4 Sternocostal external view of the heart.

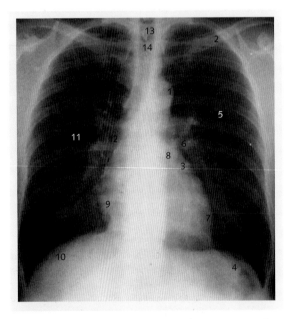

Fig. 2.3 Normal postero-anterior (PA) chest X-ray. 1, arch of aorta/aortic knuckle; 2, clavicle; 3, left atrial appendage; 4, left dome of diaphragm; 5, left lung; 6, left hilum; 7, left ventricular border; 8, pulmonary trunk; 9, right atrial border; 10, right dome of diaphragm; 11, right lung; 12, right hilum; 13, spine of vertebrae; 14, trachea.
(Courtesy of Professor Dame M Turner-Warwick, Dr M Hodson, Professor B Corrin and Dr I Kerr.)

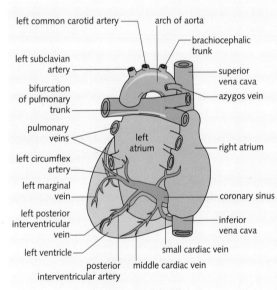

Fig. 2.5 Postero-inferior external view of the heart.

External structure of the heart

The heart lies obliquely about two-thirds to the left and one-third to the right of the median plane (Figs 2.4–2.6). It has the following surfaces:

- The base of the heart is located posteriorly and formed mainly by the left atrium.
- The apex of the heart is formed by the left ventricle and is posterior to the fifth intercostal space.

- The sternocostal surface of the heart is formed mainly by the right ventricle.
- The diaphragmatic surface is formed mainly by the left ventricle and part of the right ventricle.
- The pulmonary surface is mainly formed by the left ventricle.

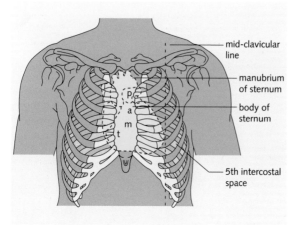

Fig. 2.6 Surface markings of the heart (a, aortic valve; m, mitral valve; p, pulmonary valve; t, tricuspid valve). These are anatomical relations – see Chapter 8 for auscultatory areas.

The heart borders of the anterior surface are as follows:

- Right: right atrium.
- Left: left ventricle and left auricle.
- Inferior: right ventricle mainly and part of left ventricle.
- Superior: right and left auricles.

HINTS AND TIPS

When examining the cardiovascular system it is important to remember that the right ventricle lies anteriorly and faces the sternocostal surface. In certain conditions causing pulmonary hypertension, the right ventricle is forced to work excessively hard, and this can be felt as a heave on the precordium.

Internal structure of the heart

The internal structure of the heart is shown in Fig. 2.7. The right atrium contains the orifices of the superior and inferior venae cavae and coronary sinus. The right ventricle is separated from the right atrium by the tricuspid (three cusps) valve. The right ventricle is separated from its outflow tract (the pulmonary trunk) by the pulmonary valve. This has three semilunar valve cusps.

The left atrium has the orifices of four pulmonary veins in its posterior wall and is separated from the left ventricle by the mitral (sometimes referred to as bi-cuspid, i.e. two cusps) valve. The left ventricle is separated from its outflow tract (the aorta) by the aortic valve, which also has three semilunar valve cusps.

> In approximately 1 % of the population, the aortic valve is bicuspid (has only two cusps). This usually goes unnoticed but puts a person at increased risk of developing aortic stenosis.

Coronary arteries

The coronary arteries are shown in Figs 2.8 and 2.9. The left coronary artery arises just distal to the left anterior cusp of the aortic valve. The right coronary artery arises from the right anterior aortic sinus just above the right anterior cusp of the aortic valve. The coronary arteries are the first branches of the aorta; the heart supplies itself with a blood supply before any other organ.

> Knowledge of the arterial supply to the myocardium is essential in determining which vessel is affected in ischaemic heart disease, and allows us to predict the sequelae of an event. Inferior infarcts caused by disease of the right coronary artery, for example, are more prone to bradyarrhythmias as this artery also supplies the sinoatrial (SA) and atrioventricular (AV) nodes.

Coronary veins

The coronary veins drain mainly into the coronary sinus, which drains directly into the right atrium (Figs 2.10 and 2.11). There are some small veins that drain directly into the heart chambers. Generally, these drain into the right side of the heart.

Great vessels

'Great vessels' is the term used to denote the large arteries and veins that are directly related to the heart. The great arteries include the pulmonary trunk and the aorta (and sometimes its three main branches: the brachiocephalic, the left common carotid and the left subclavian). The great veins include the pulmonary veins and the superior and inferior venae cavae. The great vessels and their thoracic branches are illustrated in Figs 2.12–2.14.

The vascular tree

The anatomy of the circulatory system is shown in Figs 2.15–2.27.

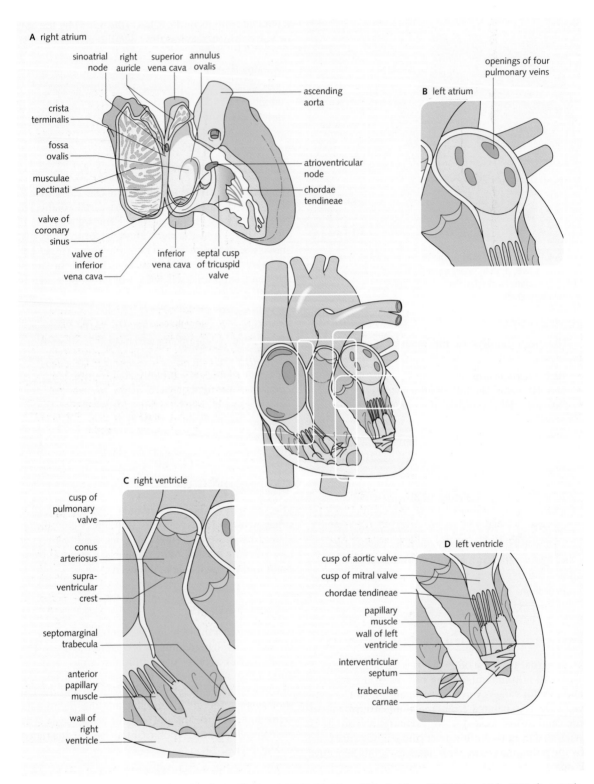

Fig. 2.7 Internal structure of the four chambers of the heart. (A) Right atrium. (B) Left atrium. (C) Right ventricle. (D) Left ventricle.

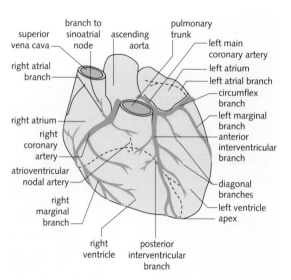

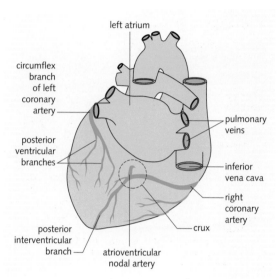

Fig. 2.8 Anterior surface of the heart showing coronary arteries. The left coronary artery has two terminal branches: the anterior interventricular branch (also called the left anterior descending artery, or 'widow's artery'). The anterior interventricular branch supplies both ventricles and the interventricular septum. The circumflex branch supplies the left atrium and the inferior part of the left ventricle. The right coronary artery supplies the sinoatrial (SA) node via the right atrial branch.

Fig. 2.9 Postero-inferior surface of the heart showing coronary arteries. The right coronary artery gives off a right marginal branch (see Fig. 2.7) and a large posterior interventricular branch. Near the apex, the posterior interventricular branch may anastomose with the anterior interventricular branch of the left coronary artery. The right coronary artery mainly supplies the right atrium, right ventricle and interventricular septum. It may also supply part of the left atrium and left ventricle. The nodal branch supplies the atrioventricular (AV) node.

Cerebrovascular disease is the most common neurological problem experienced in the Western world. It occurs as the result of clot deposition, or more rarely from a bleed, in the circle of Willis. The circle, being a complete anastomosis, allows blood to flow irrespective of a small blockage, minimizing the neurological insult of the stroke.

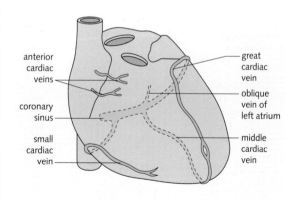

Fig. 2.10 Anterior view of the heart showing coronary veins.

DEVELOPMENT OF THE HEART AND GREAT VESSELS

The heart develops in the cardiogenic region of the mesoderm from week 3. This region is at the cranial end of the embryonic disc. Angioblastic cords (aggregates of endothelial cell precursors) develop and here they coalesce to form two lateral endocardial tubes. During week 4, these tubes fuse together to form the primitive heart tube and the heart begins to pump (Fig. 2.28).

From weeks 5 to 8, the primitive heart tube folds and remodels to form the four-chambered heart.

Initially, the primitive heart tube develops a series of expansions separated by shallow sulci (infoldings, Fig. 2.29).

The primitive atrium will give rise to parts of both future atria. The primitive ventricle will make up most of the left ventricle. The bulbus cordis will form the right ventricle. The truncus arteriosus will form the ascending aorta and the pulmonary trunk.

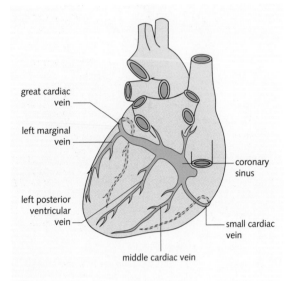

Fig. 2.11 Postero-inferior view of the heart showing coronary veins.

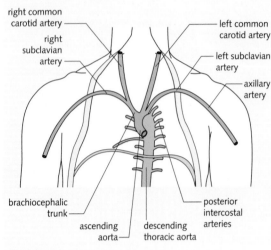

Fig. 2.12 The thoracic aorta and its branches.

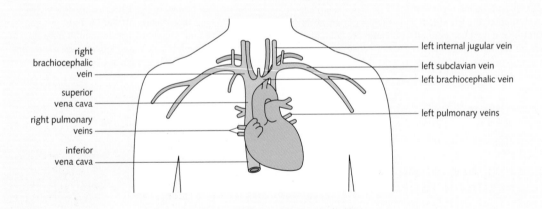

Fig. 2.13 Veins of the thorax.

HINTS AND TIPS

There are many difficult terms in embryology. Try to understand them by considering what process the term describes. For example, the septum primum is the first (*primus* means first in Latin) septum to form and septum secundum is the second septum to form.

Venous blood initially enters the sinus horns of the sinus venosus from the cardinal veins (a branch of the umbilical vein). Within the next few weeks, the whole systemic venous return is shifted to the right sinus horn through the newly formed superior and inferior venae cavae. The left sinus horn becomes the coronary sinus, which drains the myocardium.

In weeks 5–6, the septum primum and the septum secundum grow to separate the right and left atria (Fig. 2.30). These septa are incomplete and leave two openings (foramina or ostia) that allow blood to move between the atria. The septum primum grows downwards from the superior, posterior wall. The foramen (ostium primum) it creates narrows as the septum grows.

While the septum primum is growing, a thicker septum secundum also starts to form. This septum secundum does not meet the septum intermedium, leaving

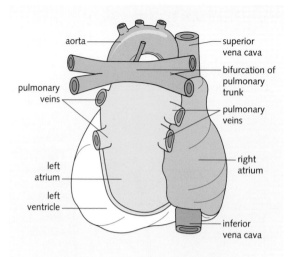

Fig. 2.14 Posterior view of the pulmonary vessels.

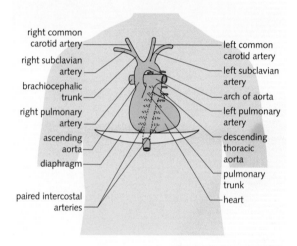

Fig. 2.15 Arterial supply of the thorax.

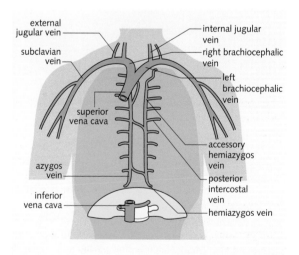

Fig. 2.16 Venous drainage of the thorax.

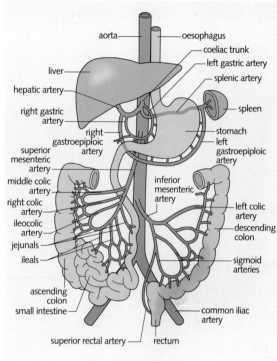

Fig. 2.17 Arterial supply of the abdomen.

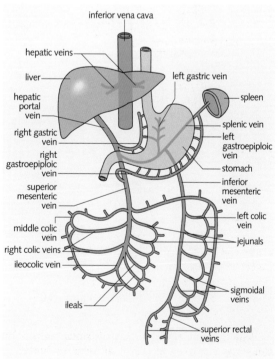

Fig. 2.18 Venous drainage of the abdomen.

an opening called the foramen ovale near the floor of the right atrium.

Blood now has to shunt from the right to the left atrium through the two staggered openings in the septum, the foramen ovale and the ostium secundum (Fig. 2.31). At birth, the two septa are fused together to abolish any foramen between the two atria.

During weeks 5–6, the atrioventricular (tricuspid and mitral) valves develop. The heart undergoes some

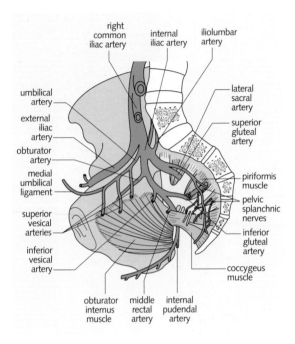

Fig. 2.19 Vessels of the pelvis.

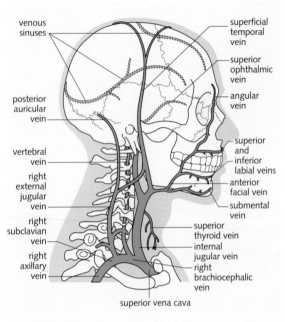

Fig. 2.21 Veins of the neck and head.

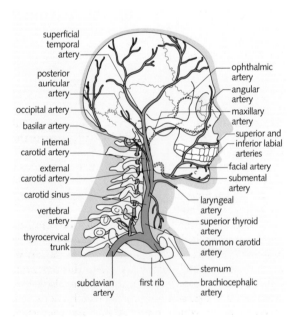

Fig. 2.20 Arteries of the neck and head.

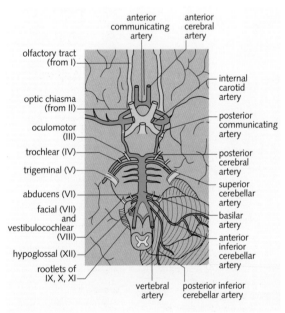

Fig. 2.22 Arteries of the brain. The circle of Willis is an anastomotic loop constructed from the anterior and posterior communicating, and anterior and posterior cerebral arteries. The cranial nerves are also shown.

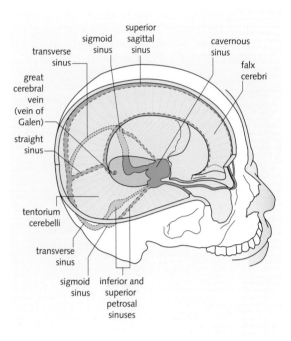

Fig. 2.23   Venous drainage of the brain.

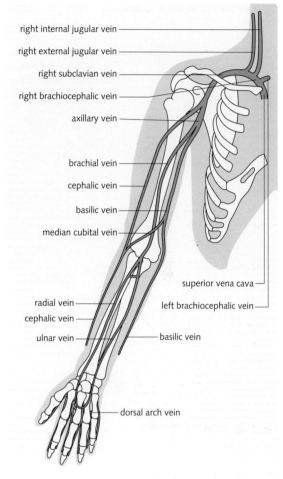

Fig. 2.25   Venous drainage of the upper limbs.

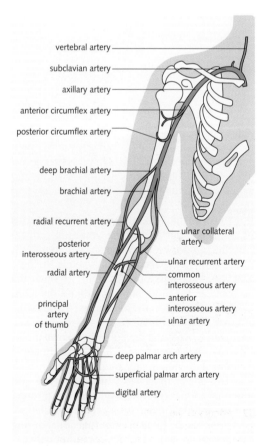

Fig. 2.24   Arterial supply of the upper limbs.

changes that bring the atria and ventricles into their correct positions and align the outflow tracks with the ventricles.

The inferior part of the bulboventricular sulcus grows into the muscular ventricular septum. Growth stops in week 7 to wait for the left outflow track to develop, leaving an interventricular foramen.

In weeks 7–8, the truncus arteriosus (the common outflow tract of the heart) is divided in two by a spiral process of central septation, which results in the formation of the aorta and pulmonary trunk. This septum is called the truncoconal septum. This septum also grows into the ventricles, and it forms the membranous ventricular septum, which joins the muscular ventricular septum. This completes the septation of the ventricles. Swellings develop at the inferior end of the truncus arteriosus, and these give rise to the arterial (pulmonary and aortic) valves.

Fig. 2.26 Arterial supply of the lower limbs.

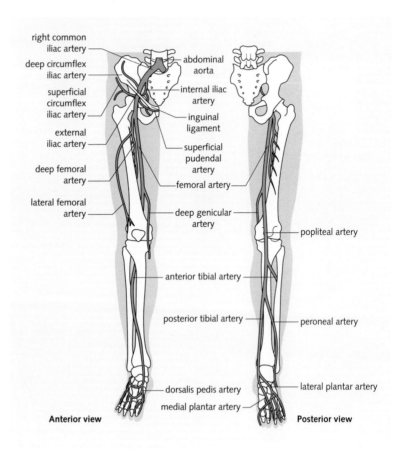

right common iliac artery
deep circumflex iliac artery
superficial circumflex iliac artery
external iliac artery
deep femoral artery
lateral femoral artery
abdominal aorta
internal iliac artery
inguinal ligament
superficial pudendal artery
femoral artery
deep genicular artery
popliteal artery
anterior tibial artery
posterior tibial artery
peroneal artery
dorsalis pedis artery
medial plantar artery
lateral plantar artery

Anterior view

Posterior view

Development of the vasculature

The vasculature develops from the angioblastic cords of mesoderm. The aortic ends of the primitive heart tube become the aortic arches and dorsal aortae. The aortic arches develop into the great arteries of the neck and thorax, whereas the dorsal aortae produce the following branches:

- Ventral branches (derived from the remnants of the vitelline arteries), which supply the gastrointestinal tract.
- Lateral branches, which supply retroperitoneal structures (e.g. kidneys).
- Intersegmental branches, which supply the rest of the body.

The paired dorsal aortae connect to the umbilical arteries, which carry blood to the placenta. The venous system consists of three components, which are initially paired:

- Cardinal system, which drains the head, neck, body wall, and limbs.
- Vitelline veins, which drain the yolk sac.
- Umbilical veins, which carry blood from the placenta to the embryo.

Initially, the venous system drains into the sinus horns, and subsequently into the venae cavae and right atrium. In general, it is the right-sided veins that persist while the left-sided veins regress during gestation, and so systemic venous drainage is via the vena cava to the right side of the heart.

Within the liver, the vitelline system forms the ductus venosus, shunting blood from the umbilical vein directly into the inferior vena cava during gestation. This is vital, as it allows oxygenated blood to enter the right atrium of the heart, pass predominantly through the foramen ovale and then be pumped around the fetus. The foramen ovale enables the oxygenated blood in the right atrium to pass into the left atrium and reach the systemic circulation, bypassing the pulmonary circulation.

The ductus arteriosus develops from the sixth aortic arch. It connects the pulmonary arteries to the descending aorta. This allows oxygenated blood pumped into the pulmonary arteries (i.e. blood not shunted through the foramen ovale) to enter the systemic circulation. This is necessary as the lungs are not functional during gestation, negating the need for a large pulmonary circulation. The duct is kept open during fetal life by

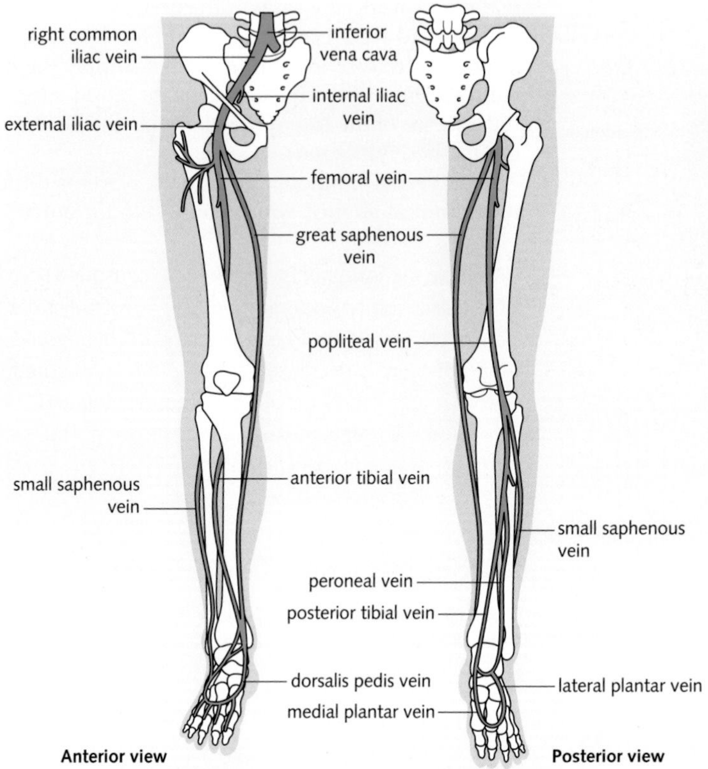

Fig. 2.27 Venous drainage of the lower limbs.

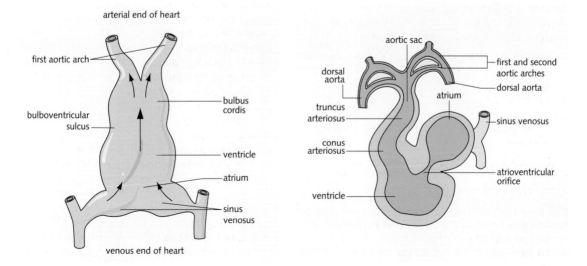

right common iliac vein

inferior vena cava

internal iliac vein

external iliac vein

femoral vein

great saphenous vein

popliteal vein

small saphenous vein

anterior tibial vein

small saphenous vein

peroneal vein

posterior tibial vein

dorsalis pedis vein

medial plantar vein

lateral plantar vein

Anterior view

Posterior view

arterial end of heart

first aortic arch

bulboventricular sulcus

bulbus cordis

ventricle

atrium

sinus venosus

venous end of heart

Fig. 2.28 Primitive heart tube at 21 days.

aortic sac

dorsal aorta

truncus arteriosus

conus arteriosus

ventricle

first and second aortic arches

dorsal aorta

atrium

sinus venosus

atrioventricular orifice

Fig. 2.29 Primitive heart tube as it folds and expands.

13

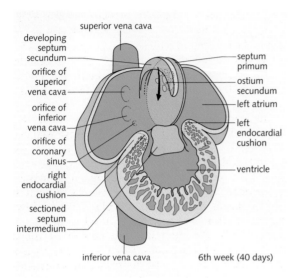

Fig. 2.30 Initial septation of the atria. The septum primum forms at day 33, and eventually leaves a hole (the ostium secundum). The septum secundum develops later, at day 40, and is deficient at the foramen ovale. (Redrawn with permission from Larsen WJ. Human embryology, 2nd edn. Edinburgh: Churchill Livingstone, 1997.)

circulating prostaglandins, and this stimulation may be continued artificially early in the neonatal period.

The head receives a preferential blood supply, so if there is a decrease in umbilical artery supply the head will continue to receive an adequate blood supply at the expense of the rest of the body (i.e. the head grows but the body does not).

Deoxygenated blood returns to the placenta through the umbilical arteries, which connect to the aorta.

Multiple measurements are taken at ultrasound scan in pregnant women, including Doppler flow studies of the umbilical vessels, and head/abdomen circumference ratio. If there is decreased arterial supply, intrauterine growth retardation (IUGR) can be predicted and monitored by serial measurements showing a failure in growth of abdominal circumference.

Circulatory adaptations at birth

A series of changes convert the single system of blood flow around the fetus into dual systems at birth (Figs 2.32 and 2.33). Blood flow in the umbilical vessels

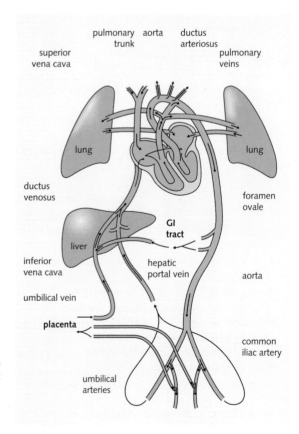

Fig. 2.31 Completed septation of the atria. The septum primum is deficient superiorly at the ostium secundum. The septum secundum is deficient inferiorly at the foramen ovale. Blood shunts from the right atrium through these two holes in the septa to the left atrium. In this way, blood bypasses the lungs in the fetal circulation. As these two openings are staggered, fusion of the septum primum and secundum will abolish any shunt between the atria. (Redrawn with permission from Larsen WJ. Human embryology, 2nd edn. Edinburgh: Churchill Livingstone, 1997.)

Fig. 2.32 Fetal circulation in utero (GI tract, gastrointestinal tract).

drop in the right atrium and a pressure rise in the left atrium (caused by an increased pulmonary venous return to the left atrium). This changes the pressure gradient across the atrial septum and forces the flexible septum primum against the rigid septum secundum, closing the foramen ovale. These two septa fuse together after about 3 months.

The ductus venosus closes soon after birth. The mechanism is unclear, but it is thought to involve prostaglandin inhibition. The closure is not vital to life, as the umbilical vein no longer carries any blood. The remnant of the ductus venosus is the ligamentum venosus.

The ductus arteriosus closes 1–8 days after birth. It is thought that as the pulmonary vascular resistance falls, the pressure drop in the pulmonary trunk causes blood to flow from the aorta into the pulmonary trunk through the ductus arteriosus. This blood is oxygenated and the increase in P_{O_2} causes the smooth muscle in the wall of the ductus to constrict dye to decreased prostaglandin production, obstructing the flow in the ductus arteriosus. Eventually, the intima of the ductus arteriosus thickens – complete obliteration of the ductus results in the formation of the ligamentum arteriosum, which attaches the pulmonary trunk to the aorta.

Congenital abnormalities

The embryological development of the heart is a complex process involving many coordinated steps. Defects arise if the process does not occur correctly. Congenital heart defects have an incidence of 6–8 per 1000 live-born infants. They may present in the first year of life, during childhood or remain asymptomatic for life. When thinking about the effects of a given congenital abnormality, it is important to consider the pressure gradients that are present within the cardiovascular system as these will determine where blood flows and for the most part allow you to understand the symptoms and signs that arise.

Left-to-right shunts

Left-to-right shunts very rarely cause cyanosis because all the blood is passing through the pulmonary circulation and being oxygenated.

Atrial septal defect

An atrial septal defect (ASD) is caused by a failure of proper closure of the foramen ovale or by a defect in the septum secundum. Blood moves from the left atrium into the right atrium because of the pressure gradient (Fig. 2.34). Atrial septal defects make up 10% of all congenital heart defects.

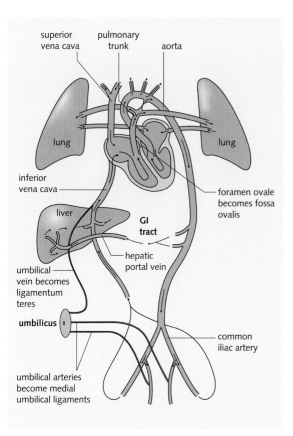

Fig. 2.33 Neonatal circulation shortly after birth. Note the closure of the foramen ovale, ductus arteriosus, ductus venosus and umbilical vessels closing off the fetal shunts (GI tract, gastrointestinal tract).

drastically declines in the first few minutes after birth because of:

- Compression of the cord.
- Vasoconstriction in response to cold, mechanical stimuli and circulating fetal catecholamines as a result of the stress of descending through the birth canal.

At birth, the pulmonary vascular resistance falls rapidly because:

- The thorax of the fetus is compressed on descent, emptying the amniotic fluid from the lungs.
- The mechanical effect of ventilation opens the constricted alveolar vessels.
- Raising P_{O_2} and lowering P_{CO_2} cause vasodilatation of the pulmonary vessels.

This produces an increase in the pulmonary blood flow.

The sudden cessation of umbilical blood flow and the opening of the pulmonary system causes a change in the pressure balance in the atria. There is a pressure

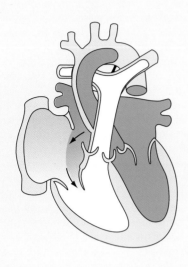

Fig. 2.34 Atrial septal defect. (Courtesy of Lissauer T, Clayden G. Illustrated textbook of paediatrics, 2nd edn. London: Mosby, 2001.)

Ventricular septal defect

A ventricular septal defect (VSD) is a failure of fusion of the interventricular septum (Fig. 2.35). Blood shunts through a hole in the interventricular septum down the pressure gradient from the left ventricle to the right ventricle. If there is a large left-to-right shunt, there will be a great deal of blood entering the right ventricle and pulmonary circulation, causing pulmonary hypertension. Eventually, the pulmonary hypertension will cause irreversible damage to the pulmonary vasculature.

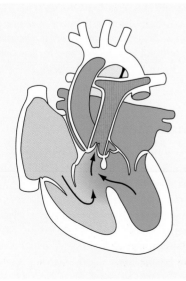

Fig. 2.35 Ventricular septal defect. (Courtesy of Lissauer T, Clayden G. Illustrated textbook of paediatrics, 2nd edn. London: Mosby, 2001.)

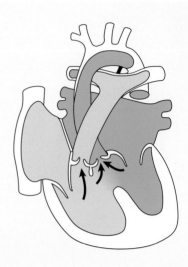

Fig. 2.36 Eisenmenger's syndrome. The shunt has reversed (and now goes from right to left). Less blood now goes into the pulmonary trunk and the patient becomes cyanosed. (Courtesy of Lissauer T, Clayden G. Illustrated textbook of paediatrics, 2nd edn. London: Mosby, 2001.)

The increased pressures in the right side of the heart may eventually lead to reversal of the shunt from right to left. This phenomenon, known as Eisenmenger's syndrome, is irreversible and causes cyanosis (Fig. 2.36).

Patent ductus arteriosus

Patent ductus arteriosus is when the ductus arteriosus fails to close, allowing communication of blood between the systemic and pulmonary circulations (Fig. 2.37). In preterm infants, the duct will ultimately close, but it can be closed with indometacin (inhibits prostaglandin production), or it may require closure with a catheter-delivered device.

When considering congenital disorders of the heart, it is important to visualize the pressure changes that occur in the cardiac cycle in order to work out which shunting mechanism and murmur occurs with each defect. For example, in a ventricular septal defect the left ventricular pressure is greater than the right because of its larger muscle mass, so, therefore, blood is going to flow from left to right. As this shunt occurs throughout systole a pansystolic murmur occurs. Cyanosis does not occur unless deoxygenated blood 'dilutes' oxygenated blood before entering the systemic circulation.

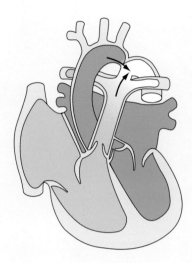

Fig. 2.37 Patent ductus arteriosus. This is often found with coarctation of the aorta (shown). It allows mixing of systemic and pulmonary blood. Movement of blood within the ductus can occur in both directions depending upon the relative pressures in the aorta and the pulmonary trunk. (Courtesy of Lissauer T, Clayden G. Illustrated textbook of paediatrics, 2nd edn. London: Mosby, 2001.)

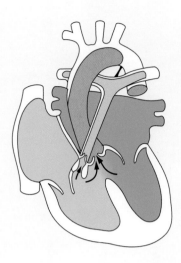

Fig. 2.38 Tetralogy of Fallot. The right-to-left shunt that results causes cyanosis. (Courtesy of Lissauer T, Clayden G. Illustrated textbook of paediatrics, 2nd edn. London: Mosby, 2001.)

Right-to-left shunts

Right-to-left shunts commonly cause cyanosis early in life. Clubbing commonly develops in cyanotic congenital heart disease.

Tetralogy of Fallot

Tetralogy of Fallot (Fig. 2.38) is a combination of:

- Large ventricular septal defect.
- Pulmonary stenosis.
- Right ventricular hypertrophy.
- Aorta overriding the interventricular septum.

Corrective surgery is required, which can be started at 4–6 months of age.

Transposition of the great arteries

Transposition of the great arteries occurs when the truncoconal septum develops, but it does not spiral (Fig. 2.39). The left ventricle pumps blood into the pulmonary trunk and the right ventricle pumps blood into the aorta creating two closed systems. There is usually also an atrial septal defect, ventricular septal defect or patent ductus arteriosus, allowing blood from the two systems to mix, otherwise this would be incompatible with life.

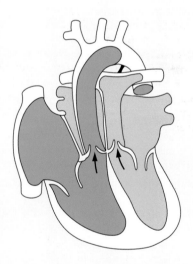

Fig. 2.39 Transposition of the great arteries. This is incompatible with life without a ventricular (VSD) or atrial septal defect (ASD) or a patent ductus arteriosus. (Courtesy of Lissauer T, Clayden G. Illustrated textbook of paediatrics, 2nd edn. London: Mosby, 2001.)

Obstructive congenital defects

Coarctation of the aorta

Coarctation of the aorta is a narrowing of the aorta around the area of the ductus arteriosus (Fig. 2.40). It is frequently associated with a ventricular septal defect or a bicuspid aortic valve and is important to consider in a young person with hypertension.

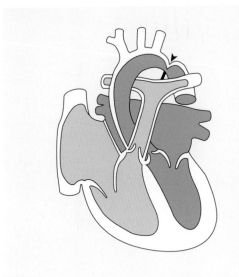

Fig. 2.40 Coarctation of the aorta, causing stenosis. (Courtesy of Lissauer T, Clayden G. Illustrated textbook of paediatrics, 2nd edn. London: Mosby, 2001.)

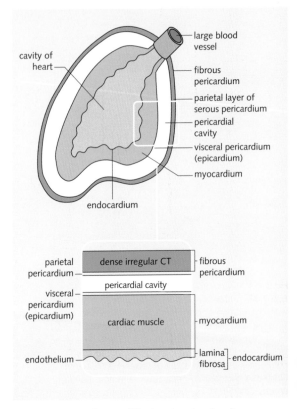

Fig. 2.41 Tissue layers of the heart and pericardium (CT, connective tissue).

HISTOLOGY

Tissue layers of the heart and pericardium (Fig. 2.41)

Pericardium

The pericardium consists of an outer fibrous pericardial sac, enclosing the whole heart, and an inner double layer of flat mesothelial cells, called the serous pericardium. The two layers of the serous pericardium are:

- The parietal pericardium, which is attached to the fibrous sac.
- The visceral pericardium, which forms part of the epicardium and which covers the heart's outer surface.

The serous pericardium produces approximately 50 mL of pericardial fluid, which sits in the pericardial cavity formed by the parietal and visceral layers. The primary function of this fluid is to provide lubrication so that the heart can move within the pericardium during the cardiac cycle.

Heart

The heart itself contains three layers:

- Epicardium.
- Myocardium.
- Endocardium.

Epicardium

The epicardium is a thin layer of connective tissue that contains adipose tissue, nerves and the coronary arteries and veins.

Myocardium

Myocardium is the thickest layer of the heart, and it is made up of cardiac muscle cells. The thickness of the myocardium is greatest in the left ventricle and smallest in the atria. All the muscle layers attach to the fibro-collagenous heart skeleton, which provides a stable base for contraction. The atrial myocardium secretes atrial natriuretic peptide (ANP) when stretched, promoting salt and water excretion. The ventricular myocardium, however, secretes brain natriuretic peptide (BNP) when stretched. While this is rather a misnomer, it is increasingly being used to monitor left ventricular dysfunction in heart failure.

Endocardium

The endocardium has three layers: an outermost connective tissue layer (which contains nerves, veins and Purkinje fibres), a middle layer of connective tissue and an endothelium of flat endothelial cells.

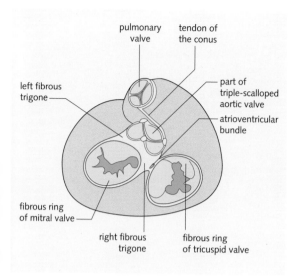

Fig. 2.42 Superior view of the heart skeleton. Vessels and external muscle layers have been removed.

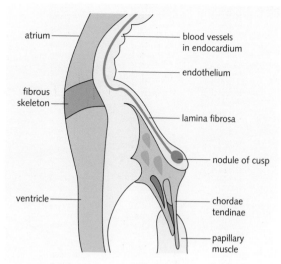

Fig. 2.43 Structure of a heart valve.

Fibrous heart skeleton

The fibrous heart skeleton consists of fibrotendinous (fibrocollagenous) rings of dense connective tissue that encircle the base of the aorta and pulmonary trunk and the atrioventricular openings (Fig. 2.42). The heart valves and cardiac muscle attach to these rings and they form a solid base on which the heart can contract. The fibrous structure also electrically insulates the atria from the ventricles. The membranous interventricular septum is a downward extension of the fibrocollagenous tissue, and it contains the bundle of His. The atrioventricular node and the bundle of His form the only conduction pathway through the skeleton in health and, therefore, the only electrical link between the atria and the ventricles. The Wolff–Parkinson–White syndrome (discussed in Ch. 3) is caused by an additional conduction pathway between the atria and ventricles.

> **HINTS AND TIPS**
>
> It is important to remember that despite being commonly referred to as the heart skeleton, it is formed from fibrous connective tissue, NOT bone.

Valves

The heart valves are avascular (i.e. they have no blood supply) (Fig. 2.43). This is important if bacteria invade the valves, because there is little immune reaction and infective endocarditis may result. Their avascular nature also means that they can be replaced with a porcine (pig) or bovine (cow) tissue valve without generating a rejection-like immune response.

Cardiac myocytes

There are three types of myocytes – work myocytes, nodal cells and conduction fibres:

- Work myocytes are the main contractile cells.
- Nodal cells make up the SA node and AV node, and generate cardiac electrical impulses.
- Conduction (Purkinje) fibres have a greater diameter than work myocytes (70–80 μm) and allow fast conduction of action potentials around the heart.

Ultrastructure of the typical cardiomyocyte

The typical cardiac myocyte (Fig. 2.44) has the following features:

- Length of 50–100 μm (shorter than skeletal muscle fibres).
- Diameter of 10–20 μm.
- Single, central nucleus.
- Branched structure.
- Attached to neighbouring cells via intercalated disks at the branch points. These cell junctions consist of desmosomes (which hold the cells together via proteoglycan bridges) and gap junctions (which allow electrical conductivity).
- Many mitochondria arranged in rows between the intracellular myofibrils.

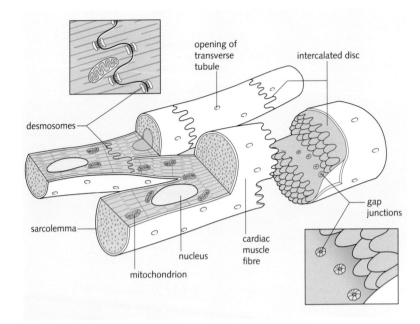

Fig. 2.44 Cardiac myocyte arrangement. Myocytes are branched, and they attach to each other through desmosomes to form muscle fibres. Gap junctions enable rapid electrical conductivity between cells. There is an extensive sarcoplasmic reticulum, which is the internal Ca^{2+} store. The contractile elements within each cell produce characteristic bands and lines. In between each myofibril unit there are rows of mitochondria. Accompanying blood vessels and connective tissue lie alongside each muscle fibre. (Redrawn with permission from Tortora GJ, Grabowski SR. Principles of anatomy and physiology, 9th edn. New York: John Wiley & Sons, 2000.)

- T (transverse) tubules organized in diads with cisternae of sarcoplasmic reticulum (Fig. 2.45), which enable rapid electrical conduction deep into the cell, activating the whole contractile apparatus.
- Extensive sarcoplasmic reticulum, which stores Ca^{2+} ions necessary for electrical activity and contraction.

Each myocyte contains many myofibril-like units (similar to the myofibrils of skeletal muscle) (Fig. 2.45). These units are made up of sarcomeres attached end-to-end and collected into a bundle. A sarcomere is the basic contractile unit. It is composed of two bands, the A band and the I band, between two Z lines.

- The A (anisotropic) band is made up of thick myosin filaments and some interdigitating actin filaments.
- The I (isotropic) band is made up of thin actin filaments that do not overlap with myosin filaments. Troponin and tropomyosin are also contained in the thin filaments.
- The Z line is a dark-staining structure containing α-actinin protein that provides attachment for the thin filaments.

STRUCTURE OF THE VESSELS

The vessels of the circulatory system can be classified anatomically or according to their function.

Anatomical classification

- Elastic arteries (e.g. aorta and common carotids).
- Muscular arteries (e.g. coronary, cerebral, and popliteal arteries).
- Arterioles.
- Capillaries.
- Postcapillary venules.
- Muscular venules.
- Veins.

Functional classification

- Conductance: elastic arteries and muscular arteries.
- Resistance: primarily arterioles.
- Exchange: capillaries.
- Capacitance: venules and veins.

All blood vessels, except capillaries and venules, have walls made up of three main layers (or tunicae):

- Tunica intima: composed of a single layer of highly specialized endothelial cells that sit on a basement membrane and a very thin layer of connective tissue.
- Tunica media: composed primarily of smooth muscle cells and elastic tissue. There is a layer of elastic tissue either side of the muscular part, the internal elastic lamina and the external elastic lamina. The tunica media is most prominent in arteries. In the

A

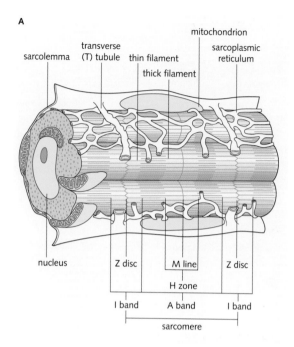

mitochondrion

transverse
sarcolemma (T) tubule thin filament sarcoplasmic
reticulum

thick filament

nucleus   Z disc   M line   Z disc

H zone

I band   A band   I band

sarcomere

B

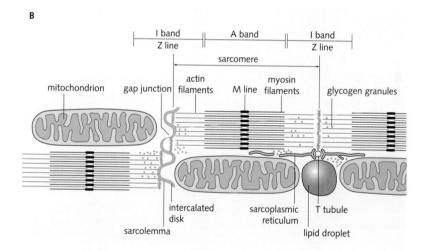

I band   A band   I band
Z line   Z line

sarcomere

actin   myosin
mitochondrion   gap junction filaments   M line filaments   glycogen granules

intercalated   sarcoplasmic   T tubule
disk   reticulum

sarcolemma   lipid droplet

Fig. 2.45 Electronmicrographic appearance of cardiac muscle. (A) Each myocyte has rows of mitochondria in between myofibril-like units. There is also an extensive sarcoplasmic reticulum and T tubule system. (B) Close-up of a myofibril-like unit shows the following bands: A band, myosin with some actin; I band, actin; Z line, attachment point for actin; M line links myosin fibres. (Reproduced with permission from [A] Williams PL (ed). Gray's anatomy, 37th edn. Edinburgh: Churchill Livingstone, 1989; [B] Davies A, Blakeley AGH, Kidd C. Human physiology. Edinburgh: Churchill Livingstone, 2001.)

elastic arteries, the elastic component is more prominent and in muscular arteries and arterioles vascular smooth muscle predominates.

- Tunica adventitia: composed of connective tissue such as collagen. Within this layer run the autonomic nerves that innervate the vascular smooth muscle. In thick walled vessels, small blood vessels called vasa vasorum are present in the adventitia,

and send penetrating branches into the media to supply the smooth muscle cells. The adventitia is the most prominent layer in veins.

Fig. 2.46 shows the relative amount of elastic, muscular and fibrous tissue in each type of vessel and Figs 2.47 and 2.48 show the structure of a generic vessel and of an elastic artery, muscular artery and a vein.

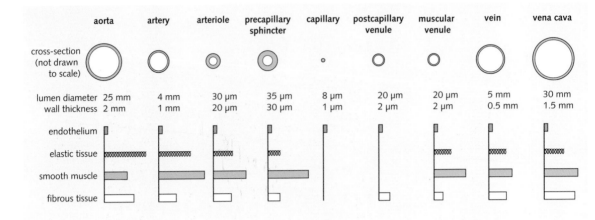

Fig. 2.46 Vessels of the circulation. (Adapted with permission from Burton AC, Physiol Rev. 34: 619, 1954).

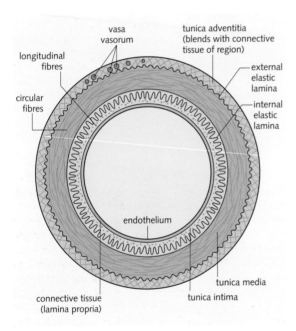

Fig. 2.47 Cross-section of a generic vessel showing the distinction between layers.

Conductance

These are low-resistance arteries with predominantly elastic walls. Their role is delivery of blood to more distal vessels, although they also have a small resistance role.

Resistance

These vessels are the small muscular arteries and arterioles, and they provide the main resistance to blood flow in the circulatory system. Resistance vessels act to control local blood flow. Dilatation of these vessels lowers resistance and increases blood flow (vasodilatation). Constriction of these vessels increases resistance and decreases blood flow (vasoconstriction). They can, therefore, influence the exchange vessels by governing the amount of blood that reaches them.

Exchange

These vessels are the numerous capillaries that have very thin walls. This optimizes their function, which is to allow rapid transfer of molecules between blood and tissues.

Capacitance

These vessels are thin-walled, low-resistance venules and veins. They act as a variable reservoir of blood and contain almost two-thirds of the blood volume. These veins are innervated by sympathetic venoconstrictor fibres which, when stimulated, constrict the veins displacing the blood back towards the heart. The presence of valves in the larger veins aids return of blood to the heart.

Compliance of capacitance vessels

In the high-pressure arterial system, the relationship between volume and pressure within the vessels is almost linear. This is not the case in the low-pressure veins and venules. At low volumes the walls of the veins are not being stretched and the veins collapse, becoming elliptical. As the volume in the vessel increases, the vein becomes round but there is very little resistance as the veins are very compliant at this stage. When they are round, any further increase in volume is met with more resistance as the inelastic wall is stretched and pressure increases quickly. Contraction of the smooth muscle within the wall of the veins reduces the compliance of the wall and there is a greater increase in pressure for a given increase in volume. This is illustrated in Fig. 2.49.

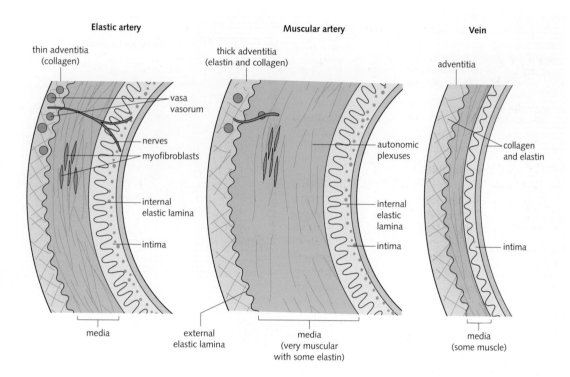

Fig. 2.48 Cross-sections through walls of elastic arteries, muscular arteries and veins.

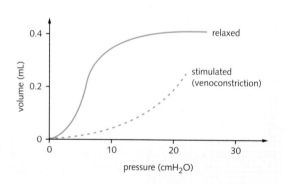

Fig. 2.49 Venous pressure curve. For a given pressure venous blood volume is greater when the venous wall muscle is relaxed than when the veins are constricted. Changes in the active wall tension can be used to displace blood into the heart.

Capillaries

The wall of a capillary is made up of a single layer of endothelial cells, which sit on a basement membrane. These thin walls are well adapted to their function as exchange vessels, providing the major site for gaseous and solute exchange between the blood and the tissues. Capillaries can be divided into two types depending on the conformation of the endothelial layer. In continuous capillaries the endothelial cells form a complete internal lining, while in fenestrated capillaries, the endothelial lining is interrupted forming pores or fenestrations, allowing passage of certain molecules. The structure of these two types of capillary is shown in Fig. 2.50.

Lymphatic vessels

The structure of a lymphatic capillary is shown in Fig. 2.51.

Endothelial cells

Endothelial cells are highly specialized and play a key role in cardiovascular function. The characteristic feature of endothelial cells on histological examination is the presence of electron-dense, ovoid organelles called Weibel–Palade bodies.

Fig. 2.50 Cross-sections of capillaries with continuous and fenestrated walls. Continuous capillary walls are less permeable than fenestrated capillary walls. (Redrawn with permission from Stevens A, Lowe J. Human histology. London: Mosby, 1997.)

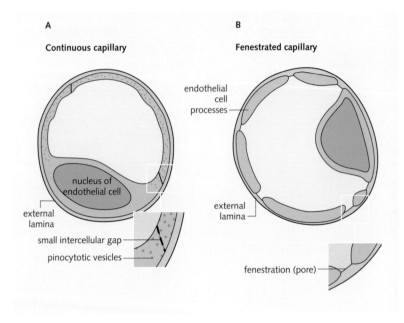

A

Continuous capillary

B

Fenestrated capillary

endothelial cell processes

nucleus of endothelial cell

external lamina

small intercellular gap

pinocytotic vesicles

external lamina

fenestration (pore)

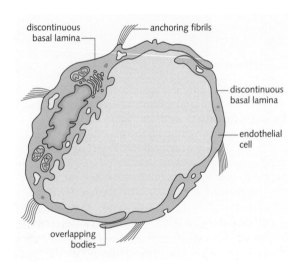

discontinuous basal lamina

anchoring fibrils

discontinuous basal lamina

endothelial cell

overlapping bodies

Fig. 2.51 Cross-section of a lymph capillary. Lymph capillaries only allow flow into the lumen but not out. Overlapping endothelial cells operate as one-way valves to accomplish this. The anchoring filaments connect the endothelial cells to the surrounding tissue. When surrounding tissues are swollen with excess interstitial fluid (e.g. in inflammation) the filaments pull the endothelial cells apart to increase lymphatic flow. The discontinuous basal lamina (basement membrane) also allows greater movement of fluids and solutes.

Endothelial cells are involved in:

- Control of vascular tone: production of various dilator and constrictor substances that act on the adjacent vascular smooth muscle tone.

- Transportation of substances between interstitium and plasma.
- Providing a friction-free surface.
- Regulation of platelet function and fibrinolysis.
- Inflammatory responses: the endothelium expresses leukocyte adhesion molecules.

Some of these functions require the secretion of a variety of substances (Fig. 2.52).

Vascular smooth muscle

Structure

The structure of vascular smooth muscle is shown in Fig. 2.53. A mass of smooth muscle functions as if it were a single unit.

Contraction of vascular smooth muscle

Contraction is initiated by a rise in intracellular $[Ca^{2+}]$. This leads to an actin–myosin interaction, which causes shortening. The process differs from that in the myocardium in the following ways:

- Myosin light chain phosphorylation: unlike skeletal or cardiac muscle, the myosin in vascular smooth muscle only becomes active if its light chains are phosphorylated. The enzyme is activated by a calcium–calmodulin complex, which is dependent on a rise in intracellular $[Ca^{2+}]$ for its formation.

Fig. 2.52 Secreted factors from endothelial cells and their functions	
Factor secreted	**Function**
Structural components	To form the basal lamina
Prostacyclin	Vasodilatation; inhibits platelet aggregation
Nitric oxide	Vasodilatation; inhibits platelet adhesion and aggregation
Angiotensin converting enzyme	Converts angiotensin I to II; degrades bradykinin and serotonin
Platelet activating factor	Activates platelets and neutrophils
Tissue plasminogen activator (tPA)	Regulates fibrinolysis
Thromboplastin	Promotes coagulation
Von Willebrand's factor	Promotes platelet adhesion and clotting

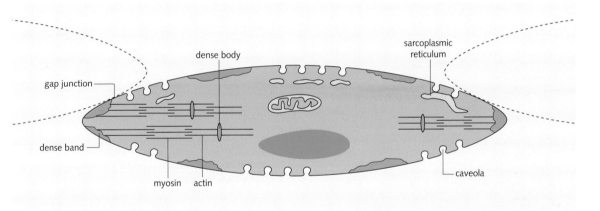

Fig. 2.53   Structure of a smooth muscle cell. The actin–myosin filaments have been magnified. (Adapted from Levick R. Introducing cardiovascular physiology. Butterworth-Heinemann, 1995. Reproduced by permission of Edward Arnold Ltd.)

- Sustained actin–myosin interactions enable vascular smooth muscle to maintain tension for 0.3% of the energy needed by skeletal muscle. The actin–myosin interactions are long-lasting because of slow myosin kinetics.

Effect of sympathetic innervation

Fig. 2.54 shows the mechanism of sympathetic innervation.

Vascular smooth muscle relaxation

Vascular smooth muscle relaxation can be brought about by three different mechanisms. Each mechanism relies upon reducing intracellular $[Ca^{2+}]$:

- Hyperpolarization: hyperpolarizing the resting membrane reduces the number of open Ca^{2+} channels, leading to a decrease in intracellular Ca^{2+} concentration and relaxation.
- Cyclic adenosine monophosphate (cAMP)-mediated vasodilatation (Fig. 2.55).
- Cyclic guanosine monophosphate (cGMP)-mediated vasodilatation (Fig. 2.56).

There are a number of small vessels (vasa nervorum) which supply nerves in the body. In certain conditions, such as diabetes, these vessels are targeted. As such, the nerves become damaged and a neuropathy develops. The neuropathy then predisposes to subsequent joint damage and ulceration

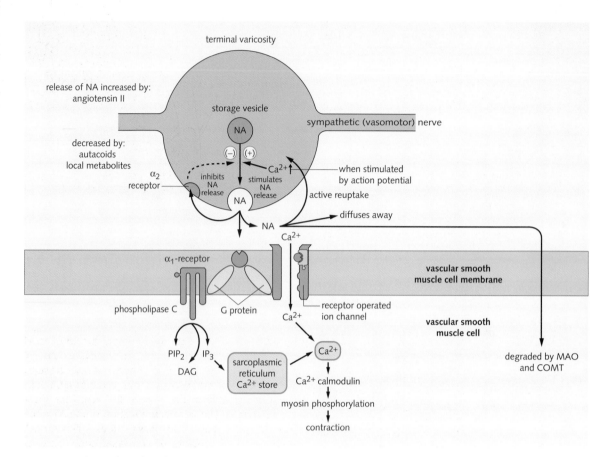

Fig. 2.54 Release of noradrenaline (NA)/norepinephrine from a sympathetic junction and its effect on the vascular smooth muscle (VSM) cell. Sympathetic stimulation results in the release of NA from the sympathetic terminal varicosities. NA acts on (among others) α_1-receptors on the VSM cells. This results in an increase in intracellular Ca^{2+} by directly opening Ca^{2+} channels and via a second messenger system releasing Ca^{2+} from the sarcoplasmic reticulum. It is the increase of intracellular Ca^{2+} that brings about contraction (AP, action potential; COMT, catechol-O-methyltransferase; DAG, diacylglycerol; IP$_3$, inositol triphosphate; MAO, monoamine oxidase; PIP$_2$, phosphatidyl inositol bisphosphate).

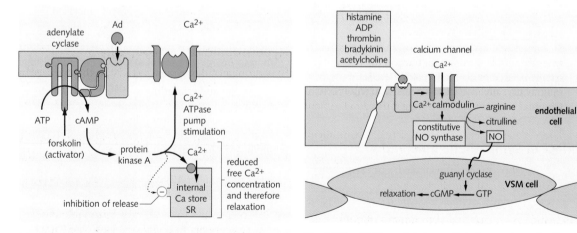

Fig. 2.55 cAMP-mediated vasodilatation as shown by the action of adrenaline (Ad)/epinephrine (ATP, adenosine triphosphate; SR, sarcoplasmic reticulum).

Fig. 2.56 cGMP-mediated vasodilatation as shown by the action of vasoactive mediators (ADP, adenosine diphosphate; GTP, guanosine triphosphate; NO, nitric oxide; VSM cell, vascular smooth muscle cell).

Cardiac electrophysiology and arrhythmia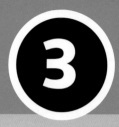

INTRODUCTION

Unlike skeletal muscle, the heart possesses intrinsic electrical activity and does not require nervous input to initiate contraction. This activity originates at the sino-atrial (SA) node, a cluster of specialized myocytes that depolarize spontaneously, often referred to as the pacemaker of the heart. Cardiomyocytes can be broadly divided into two categories in terms of their electrophysiological behaviour and function, and the appearance of their action potentials:

- Fast depolarizing cells such as atrial and ventricular myocardial cells, and cells of the His–Purkinje system. These are often referred to as work myocytes.
- Slow depolarizing cells such as those forming the SA node and atrioventricular (AV) node. These are often referred to as pacemaker cells or nodal cells.

THE CONDUCTION SYSTEM

In order for the heart to function effectively, the electrical impulse/action potential generated by the SA node must propagate through the heart in a coordinated manner. This is facilitated by a specialized conduction system (Fig. 3.1), and the presence of low resistance gap junctions, which allow direct spread of depolarization between adjacent cells. Thus the heart is often referred to as an electrical (functional) syncytium. The SA node is located in the posterior wall of the right atrium at the junction with the superior vena cava. From the SA node, the impulse passes through the atrial myocardium to the AV node, where conduction is delayed

by approximately 100 ms to allow completion of atrial contraction before depolarizing the ventricles. The AV node, located at the top of the interventricular septum, is the only point where current can pass through the fibrous skeleton from the atria to the ventricles (in a healthy heart). The secondary function of the AV node is as a backup pacemaker in situations when the SA node ceases to function or communication between the SA node and AV node is interrupted. The impulse then enters the bundle of His, which splits into right and left bundle branches. The left bundle branch then splits once again into an anterior and a posterior hemifascicle. These bundles give off fine fibres composed of specialized cardiomyocytes called Purkinje fibres that penetrate into the ventricular myocardium.

HINTS AND TIPS

It is important to remember that the cells comprising the conduction systems are specialized cardiac muscle cells, NOT nerves.

RESTING MEMBRANE POTENTIAL

The electrical potential across a plasma membrane is determined by two main factors:
- The distribution of ions across the membrane.
- The selective permeability of the cell membrane.

In cardiomyocytes, K^+ (potassium) ions are the major determinant of resting membrane potential because large numbers of K^+ channels are open constitutively.

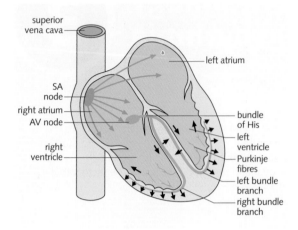

Fig. 3.1 Cardiac conduction pathway. The action potential is initiated in the sinoatrial (SA) node and spreads throughout both atria. It travels through the atrioventricular (AV) node, where it is delayed, and then to the bundle of His. From here it travels down the left and right bundle branches and into Purkinje fibres. The action potential is then spread throughout the ventricles.

These 'leak' K^+ channels mean that permeability to K^+ is high and there is a constant efflux of K^+, referred to as the 'outward background current'. The resting membrane is only slightly permeable to Na^+ (sodium), one-fortieth that of K^+, and because both the electrical and chemical gradients favour inward movement of Na^+ ions, there is a very small inward Na^+ current, which is often referred to as the 'inward background current'. The intracellular and extracellular concentrations of these ions (Fig. 3.2) are maintained by the activity of the Na^+/K^+ATPase on the sarcolemmal membrane.

A fixed negative charge is present inside cells due to the presence of intracellular proteins. This negative charge attracts K^+ ions into the cell down an electrical gradient while K^+ is simultaneously driven out of the cell down its concentration gradient. If the membrane was exclusively permeable to K^+, the resting membrane potential at equilibrium could be predicted by the Nernst equation:

$$E_K = -65 \log\left([K^+]_{out}/[K^+]_{in}\right)$$

This would result in a membrane potential of -90 mV, the equilibrium potential of K^+. In reality, because of the presence of the background inward Na^+ current through slow Na^+ channels, the true resting membrane potential in cardiomyocytes is approximately -80 mV. This is not the case in the nodal cells where it is approximately -60 mV (explained below).

CARDIAC ACTION POTENTIAL

An action potential is a transient depolarization of the cell membrane. Action potentials are initiated when the membrane is depolarized (i.e. becomes less negative)

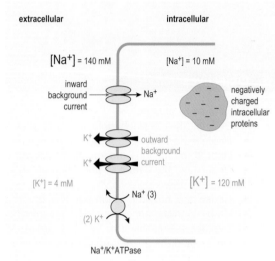

Fig. 3.2 Ion distribution and movement across the resting plasma membrane. Intracellular and extracellular concentrations of sodium [Na^+] and potassium [K^+] are shown. These concentrations are maintained by the action of the Na^+/K^+ATPase.

to a threshold potential, which can occur spontaneously (in nodal cells) but is usually stimulated by transmission from adjacent myocytes through gap junctions.

Fast cell action potential

Action potentials in fast depolarizing cells (Fig. 3.3) occur in five phases (0–4, described below) and are initiated by an action potential in an adjacent cell. The shape of the action potential is not uniform throughout work myocytes in different regions of the heart, and the speed at which action potentials are conducted also varies (Fig. 3.5).

- **Phase 0: rapid depolarization** (upstroke). When the membrane is depolarized to threshold potential (between -60 and -65 mV), fast voltage-gated Na^+ channels open, allowing rapid influx of Na^+ down its electrochemical gradient, which drives the membrane potential towards the Na^+ equilibrium potential ($+70$ mV) and causes depolarization. The rapidity of this depolarization is due to a positive feedback effect in which depolarization causes opening of additional voltage-gated Na^+ channels, causing further depolarization.
- **Phase 1: initial repolarization.** As the membrane potential reaches around $+20$ mV, the voltage-gated Na^+ channels become inactivated (self-inactivation), terminating the rapid inward Na^+ current. As this occurs, the persistent outward background K^+ current causes a slight repolarization. Phase 1 is most prominent in the Purkinje fibres.

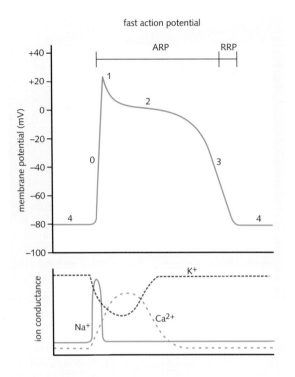

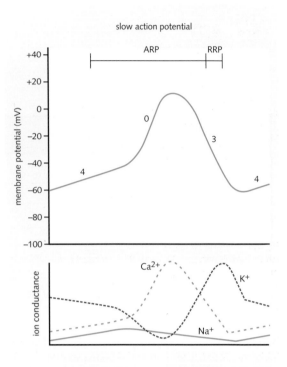

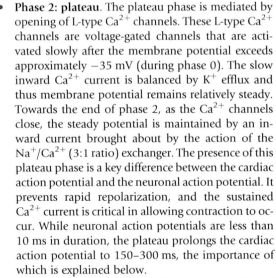

Fig. 3.3 Fast cell action potential. The phases of the action potential (0–4) are shown. Changes in membrane ion conductance throughout the action potential are shown below. (ARP, absolute refractory period; RRP, relative refractory period).

Fig. 3.4 Slow cell action potential. The phases of the action potential (0–4) are shown. Changes in membrane ion conductance throughout the action potential are shown below (ARP, absolute refractory period; RRP, relative refractory period).

- **Phase 2: plateau.** The plateau phase is mediated by opening of L-type Ca^{2+} channels. These L-type Ca^{2+} channels are voltage-gated channels that are activated slowly after the membrane potential exceeds approximately -35 mV (during phase 0). The slow inward Ca^{2+} current is balanced by K^+ efflux and thus membrane potential remains relatively steady. Towards the end of phase 2, as the Ca^{2+} channels close, the steady potential is maintained by an inward current brought about by the action of the Na^+/Ca^{2+} (3:1 ratio) exchanger. The presence of this plateau phase is a key difference between the cardiac action potential and the neuronal action potential. It prevents rapid repolarization, and the sustained Ca^{2+} current is critical in allowing contraction to occur. While neuronal action potentials are less than 10 ms in duration, the plateau prolongs the cardiac action potential to 150–300 ms, the importance of which is explained below.
- **Phase 3: repolarization.** Following termination of the inward Ca^{2+} current, additional K^+ channels open (including voltage-gated and ATP-gated), increasing K^+ efflux. This brings about repolarization of the membrane to its resting potential. A delay or

defect in the opening of these K^+ channels caused by a genetic defect delays repolarization and manifests as a long Q-T syndrome.
- **Phase 4: resting potential.**
  When repolarization is complete the membrane potential is restored to its resting value and the cycle repeats when stimulated by an adjacent cell.

Slow cell action potential (Fig. 3.4)

The cells of the SA node and AV node (nodal cells) do not have a stable resting membrane potential. The relatively lower density of constitutively open leak K^+ channels on these cells compared to fast depolarizing cells/work myocytes causes the initial resting potential in these cells to be approximately -60 mV. This membrane potential decays (depolarizes) slowly until it reaches its threshold potential at around -40 mV, when an action potential is triggered spontaneously. This decaying potential is a result of a gradual, spontaneous reduction in the K^+ permeability, reducing K^+ efflux, along with a gradual increase in Na^+ and Ca^{2+} influx through slow channels. This unstable pacemaker potential (phase 4) means that if an action potential is

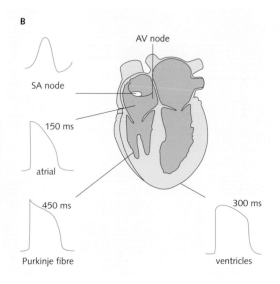

Fig. 3.5 (A) Fibre diameter and conduction velocity of the different cardiac cells. (B) Action potentials in different cardiac myocytes (SA, sinoatrial).

A

Fibre size diameter and conduction velocity		
Muscle cell (myocyte)	Diameter (mm)	Conduction velocity (m/s)
Atrial work cell	10	1
AV node	3	0.05
Purkinje fibres	75	4
Ventricular work cell	10–20	1

not stimulated by depolarization transmitted from an adjacent cell, an action potential occurs spontaneously.

Nodal cells do not express functional fast voltage-gated Na^+ channels and the upstroke of the action potential (phase 0) is produced by a slow inward Ca^{2+} current through L-type Ca^{2+} channels. As a result, the upstroke of the nodal action potential is much slower than that of the fast cells. The relatively higher threshold potential in these nodal cells is due to the fact that the L-type Ca^{2+} channels are activated at higher voltage than the fast voltage-gated Na^+ channels. After the upstroke, K^+ channels open and the resulting outward K^+ current brings about repolarization (phase 3). The action potential in nodal cells lacks the plateau phase exhibited by fast depolarizing cells.

Refractory period

During an action potential, cardiac cells are refractory to excitation, i.e. another action potential cannot be generated. There are two different refractory periods:

- Absolute refractory period, during which another action potential cannot be elicited, no matter how great the stimulus.
- Relative refractory period, during which an action potential can be initiated only if the stimulus is strong.

The two are shown in Figs 3.3 and 3.4. The absolute refractory period begins at the onset of phase 0 and lasts until the membrane has repolarized to approximately −50 mV. This refractory period is crucial as it prevents a new action potential being initiated during the previous one, allowing adequate time for ventricular filling

before the next contraction. The absolute refractory period in ventricular myocytes is approximately 250 ms in a healthy heart, thus the maximum rate the heart can beat in a coordinated manner is 240 bpm.

When the potential falls below −50 mV, some of the fast voltage-gated Na^+ channels are reset and primed to be activated again; however, only a small number are primed so a large stimulus is required. This is the so-called relative refractory period, which, in work myocytes, lasts until resting membrane potential is reached and can persist into phase 4 in nodal cells.

Control of heart rate

Nodal cells, as well as some cells in the His–Purkinje system, have the ability to depolarize spontaneously. In nodal cells, the rate at which spontaneous depolarization occurs depends on the slope of the pacemaker potential, i.e. how long it takes to reach the threshold potential after repolarization. Both the SA and AV nodes are innervated by sympathetic and parasympathetic fibres which each exert opposing chronotropic stimuli (effects on heart rate) by altering the slope of the pacemaker potential. In a denervated heart, the SA node spontaneously depolarizes at a rate of approximately 100 bpm and the AV node at between 30 and 50 bpm. Thus under normal circumstances the SA node is the dominant pacemaker and determines heart rate. If the SA node ceases to function, or conduction from the SA node to the AV node is interrupted, the AV node becomes the dominant pacemaker.

Sympathetic fibres release noradrenaline/norepinephrine, which acts on β_1 receptors, increasing the

A
symphatinic → NA → B$_1$ receptor → ↑pNa$^+$ + ↑pCa^{2+}

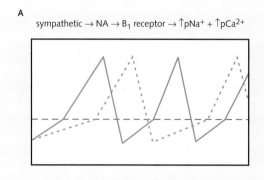

B
parasympathetic → Ach → M2 receptor → ↑pK$^+$

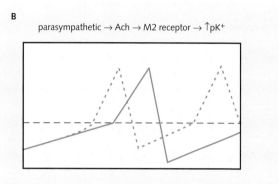

Fig. 3.6 Autonomic influences on the nodal action potential. (A) Sympathetic stimulation increases the slope of the pacemaker potential by acting on β$_1$ adrenoceptors and increasing Na$^+$ and Ca^{2+} permeability. (B) Parasympathetic stimulation decreases the slope of the pacemaker potential and hyperpolarizes the plasma membrane by acting on M2 receptors and increasing K$^+$ permeability. Dotted lines represent baseline trace, solid lines represent potential after given alteration in autonomic activity (NA, noradrenaline/norepinephrine; ACh, acetylcholine).

permeability of the nodal cell plasma membrane to Na$^+$ and Ca^{2+}, increasing the slope of the pacemaker potential. This causes an increased firing rate of the SA node, increasing heart rate, and decreases the conduction delay at the AV node.

Parasympathetic fibres release acetylcholine, which acts on muscarinic M2 receptors, increasing the permeability to K$^+$ and decreasing the Na$^+$ and Ca^{2+} permeability. This decreases the slope of the pacemaker potential, decreasing heart rate. In addition, increased parasympathetic activity causes a slight hyperpolarization at the end of each action potential, increasing the amount of depolarization that must occur before threshold potential is reached, further decreasing heart rate.

Under resting conditions, parasympathetic influences on the SA node via the vagus nerve predominate, resulting in a resting heart rate of approximately 70 bpm. The effects of autonomic innervation on the action potential in the SA and AV nodes are shown in Fig. 3.6.

EXCITATION CONTRACTION COUPLING

Excitation contraction coupling (Fig. 3.7) is the process that couples an action potential with contraction in cardiac muscle, a process underpinned by an increase in

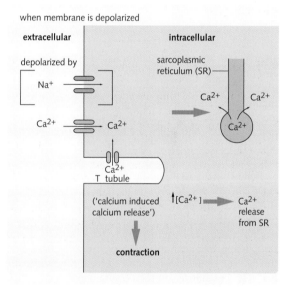

Fig. 3.7 Excitation and its effect on the myocyte (SR, sarcoplasmic reticulum).

cytosolic Ca^{2+} concentration ([Ca^{2+}]). During the plateau phase of the cardiac action potential (phase 2), Ca^{2+} enters the cytosol through the L-type Ca^{2+} channels. This influx of extracellular Ca^{2+} then stimulates further release from the sarcoplasmic reticulum (SR), a process termed Ca^{2+} induced Ca^{2+} release. Approximately 20% of the increase in cytosolic Ca^{2+} is thought to be from the extracellular space with the remainder from the SR. Once in the cytosol, Ca^{2+} ions bind troponin C, altering the position of tropomyosin and exposing the myosin heads so they can bind actin filaments, allowing contraction to take place. The greater the increase in cytosolic [Ca^{2+}], the greater the number of

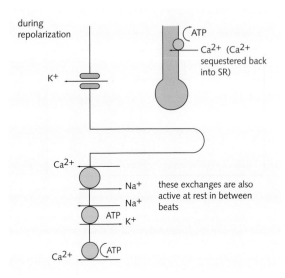

Fig. 3.8 Ion exchanges that take place during relaxation (SR, sarcoplasmic reticulum).

actin–myosin cross-bridges that are formed, and the greater the strength of contraction. Therefore, the amount of Ca^{2+} entry and thus the degree to which cytosolic $[Ca^{2+}]$ increases determines the contractility of the myocyte. Contractility is defined as the force generated by cardiac muscle for a given fibre length. Factors that influence contractility are termed inotropic factors and can have a positive or negative effect. These are described in more detail in Chapter 4.

Following myocyte contraction, it is crucial that there is an efficient system for rapidly reducing the cytosolic $[Ca^{2+}]$ to bring about relaxation and allow ventricular filling during diastole (Fig. 3.8). The Ca^{2+}ATPase on the SR is activated by increased cytosolic $[Ca^{2+}]$ and pumps approximately 80–90% of the Ca^{2+} back into the SR. The remainder is removed from the cell by the Na^+/Ca^{2+} exchanger on the plasma membrane, which utilizes the Na^+ gradient created by the activity of the Na^+/K^+ATPase to remove Ca^{2+} from the cell. Factors affecting this process can also exert inotropic effects.

ELECTROCARDIOGRAPHY

The electrocardiogram (ECG) is a recording of the electrical activity of the heart, obtained by measuring the changes in electrical potential difference across the body surface. It is usually the first investigation used to diagnose arrhythmias and the underlying cause of chest pain.

As a wave of depolarization spreads through the myocardium there will be, at any one moment, areas of myocardium that have been excited and areas that have not yet been excited. As a result, there is a difference in potential between them: one area is negatively charged (excited), the other is positive (not excited), with respect to the charge in the extracellular space. These areas can be thought of as two electrical poles that comprise the cardiac dipole. This dipole depends on both the size of the charge (which depends on the amount of muscle excited) and the direction the wave of depolarization is travelling in. In the absence of electrical activity in the heart and skeletal muscle, the electrical potential across the surface of the body is uniformly positive. The cardiac dipole (electrical activity in the heart) alters the electrical potential across the body, and by placing electrodes in certain positions, the cardiac dipole and other changes in potential can be measured in different directions. This provides the basis for electrocardiography.

Fig. 3.9 depicts how a wave of depolarization affects the potential difference between two electrodes and thus how this is translated onto an ECG trace. Remember that as the dipole has both charge (amplitude) and direction, the shape of the ECG varies depending upon the position of the recording electrode. As current travels towards the positive electrode, there is an upward deflection of the ECG waveform. As the current travels towards the negative electrode (or away from the positive one) there is a downward deflection of the ECG waveform. If current is moving perpendicular to the recording pair of electrodes there is a biphasic waveform.

Conventionally, the ECG is recorded using 12 leads (Fig. 3.10). Note that the term 'lead' is used to denote the direction in which the potential is measured and not a physical electrode – only nine electrodes are used to produce the 12 leads. The additional three lead traces are produced using the 'standard leads', which show the potential difference between specific pairs of electrodes. These leads allow us to view the direction and magnitude of electrical activity in both the frontal and transverse planes, and in any direction in these planes.

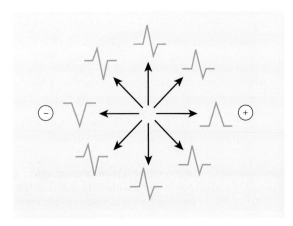

Fig. 3.9 The influence of the direction of depolarization on the ECG trace. Repolarization produces a deflection in the opposite direction.

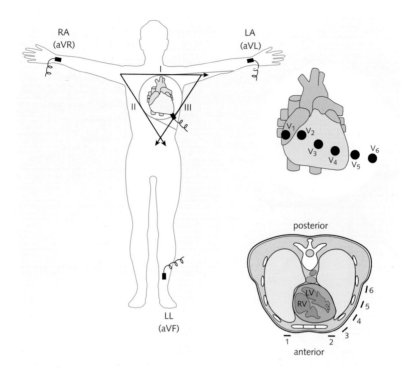

Fig. 3.10   Placement of electrocardiographic electrodes. The electrodes on the right arm (RA), left arm (LA), and left leg (LL) give the electrocardiogram trace for the frontal leads (i.e. I, II, III, aVL, aVR and aVF). Einthoven's triangle around the heart is shown. Anterior chest lead placement is shown in the frontal and transverse planes. V_1 is placed in the fourth intercostal space on the right sternal edge, and V_2 on the left sternal edge. V_4 is placed in the fifth intercostal space in the mid-clavicular line, V_5 in the anterior axillary line, and V_6 in the mid-axillary line. V_3 is placed between V_2 and V_4 (RV, right ventricle; LV, left ventricle).

Bipolar limb leads

The potential difference shown by these leads is conventionally measured from:

- Lead I: right arm (aVR) to left arm (aVL); left arm positive.
- Lead II: right arm (aVR) to left leg (aVF); left leg positive.
- Lead III: left arm (aVL) to left leg (aVF); left leg positive.

These bipolar limb leads view the heart in the frontal plane. These three leads make up Einthoven's triangle around the heart.

Unipolar limb leads

Unipolar leads measure any positive potential difference directed towards their solitary positive electrode from an estimate of zero potential. They include aVL, aVR and aVF. They also view the heart in the frontal plane.

Chest leads

Six chest electrodes labelled V_1 to V_6 measure any potential changes in the transverse plane, and they are arranged around the left side of the chest. These are also unipolar leads.

ECG traces from each of the limb leads and chest leads are shown in Figs 3.11 and 3.12 respectively.

Normal electrocardiogram

The classic ECG trace is shown in Fig. 3.13. The elements of an ECG are:

- P wave: due to atrial depolarization.
- PR interval: from the onset of the P wave to the onset of the QRS complex (approximately 120–200 ms). This represents the time taken for depolarization to propagate through the atria and the impulse to conduct through the AV node to the bundle of His.
- QRS complex: due to ventricular depolarization and is usually less than 100 ms in duration. The definitions of each wave within the QRS complex are depicted in Fig. 3.14.
- ST segment: coincides with the plateau phase of the ventricular action potential and ventricular contraction. It is usually isoelectric (flat) as the ventricles are depolarized throughout.
- T wave: due to ventricular repolarization.

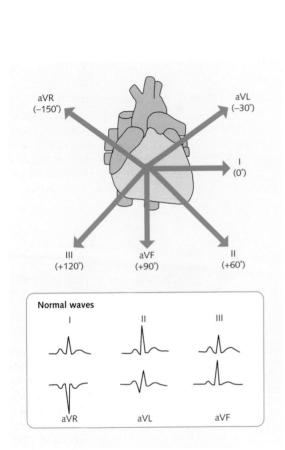

Fig. 3.11 Lead directions in the anterior plane. (Redrawn with permission from Epstein O et al. Clinical examination, 2nd edn. New York: Mosby International, 1997.)

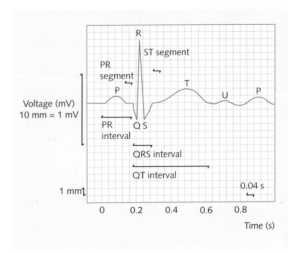

Fig. 3.13 Normal electrocardiogram trace.

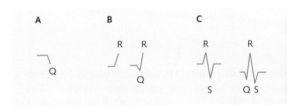

Fig. 3.14 Definitions of the ECG waves. If the wave following the P wave is negative, it is a Q wave (A). If a positive deflection follows the P wave, it is called an R wave, whether it is preceded by a Q wave or not (B). Any following negative deflection is known as an S wave, whether there has been a preceding Q wave or not (C). Abnormally large Q waves have an additional pathological significance and indicate a previous myocardial infarction.

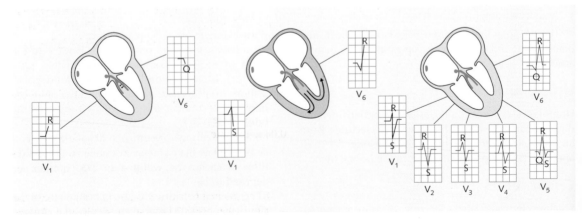

Fig. 3.12 The different anterior chest leads show different QRS traces due to the changing directions of the electrical activity. Lead V_4 is usually over the interventricular septum, and therefore usually shows equal R and S waves. Note the changing relative heights of Q, R, and S waves between leads. The changing height of the R wave from V_1 to V_6 is known as 'R wave progression'.

Why the T wave is in the same direction as the R wave

After travelling through the atria, the wave of depolarization travels from the AV node down to the apex of the heart. This is the cause of the R wave in the ECG. If repolarization of the heart then took place in the same direction the T wave would be in the opposite direction to the R wave. However, repolarization actually takes place from the apex of the heart towards the top of the septum due to differences in the duration of action potentials (shorter at the apex). Thus, the wave of repolarization occurs in the opposite direction to the wave of depolarization, and so the T wave is upright. This is a double negative: repolarization is negative depolarization and it occurs in a negative direction, so it appears as if it is positive.

Cardiac axis

The average direction of the wave of depolarization is the electrical axis of the heart, usually referred to as the cardiac axis (Fig. 3.15). This usually lies closest to lead II but is within normal limits if between $-30°$ and $+90°$. Any deviation from this range is referred to as right or left axis deviation. Right axis deviation can be caused by right ventricular hypertrophy and left axis deviation by left ventricular hypertrophy. When interpreting an ECG, it must be established whether this is normal or not.

When the depolarization wave in the ventricles is moving towards a lead, then the R wave will be larger than the S wave in that lead. When the ventricular depolarization wave is moving away from a lead, then the S wave will be larger than the R wave in that lead. If the S wave and R wave are equal then the depolarization is moving (on average) at right angles to that lead. The simplest way to assess the cardiac axis is to look at leads I and II. If the overall deflection in leads I and II is positive, then the axis is normal. If lead I is positive and II negative, it is left axis deviation. If lead I is negative and II is positive, then it is right axis deviation. If both are negative, check you have the leads on correctly!

Anterior chest leads (V_1–V_6)

The anterior chest leads look at the chest in the horizontal (or transverse) plane. The wave of depolarization in the ventricles starts in the septum and then spreads into the left and right ventricles (Fig. 3.12). Because the left ventricle is usually larger than the right, the average depolarization heads towards the left ventricle. This means that V_1 and V_2 will have a predominant S wave (i.e. negative deflection) and a small R wave, while V_5 and V_6 will have a predominant R wave (i.e. positive deflection) with a small S wave. The interventricular septum lies where there are equal positive and negative deflections (i.e. R and S waves), and is usually at V_3 or V_4. This steady increase in the size of the R wave is sometimes termed R wave progression. If this is normal then there is said to be 'good' R wave progression.

Assessment of rate

The paper speed is usually 25 mm/s, which means that in 1 second the paper has moved by five large squares (i.e. 0.2 s per large square). Every small square represents 0.04 s. The rate can be measured in a variety of ways:

- Divide 300 by the number of large squares between QRS complexes. That will give you a rate in beats per minute (bpm).
- If the interval between R waves is 1 large square the rate is 300 bpm; 2 large squares, 150 bpm; 3 large squares, 100 bpm; 4 large squares, 75 bpm; 5 large squares, 60 bpm; 6 large squares, 50 bpm (i.e. divide 300 by the number of large squares between beats).

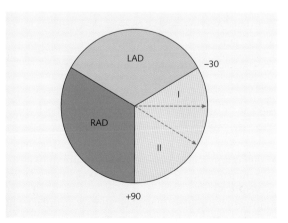

Fig. 3.15 Cardiac axis (LAD, left axis deviation; RAD, right axis deviation).

Assessment of rhythm

This is usually achieved by looking at lead II, but looking at V_1 is also helpful, as P waves cannot always be seen in lead II. Note whether the distance between the R wave peaks is consistent. If it is not, try and establish whether it is regularly irregular or irregularly irregular.

> **HINTS AND TIPS**
>
> When reading an ECG it is helpful to have a systematic approach to ensure no abnormalities are missed. Below is an example of such an approach but with experience you may develop your own system:
> - Name, age, and sex of the patient.
> - Date and time the electrocardiogram was taken.
> - Rate.
> - Rhythm.
> - Axis.
>   Next, note any abnormalities and in which lead they occur:
> - P waves: width and height.
> - PR interval.
> - QRS complex: width and height.
> - QT interval.
> - ST segment: elevated? depressed?
> - T waves: negative/positive and height.

The ECG trace can also be affected by disturbances in plasma ion concentrations:
- Hyperkalaemia: tall T, wide QRS, absent P.
- Hypokalaemia: prolonged QT interval, small T, U wave.
- Hypercalcaemia: short QT interval.
- Hypocalcaemia: long QT interval.

ARRHYTHMIA

Definitions and classification

An arrhythmia is any deviation from the heart's normal sinus rhythm. Arrhythmias may go unnoticed by the patient but can cause palpitation (an awareness of one's own heart beat) or even sudden death. ECG traces of all the arrhythmias described below are shown in Figs 3.16–3.18. Arrhythmias can be classified in a number of ways, including:

- Tachyarrhythmia (>100 bpm) OR bradyarrhythmia (<60 bpm).

First degree block (constantly prolonged PR interval)

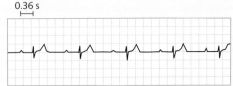
0.36 s

Each QRS complex has a preceding P wave, but the PR interval is 0.36 s (normal is 0.12–0.21 s), which is prolonged

Second degree block (Mobitz type II) (PR interval constant, but some P waves have no QRS)

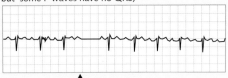

There is a constant, normal PR interval, but there are isolated P waves without following QRS complexes

Second degree block (Mobitz type I, Wenkebach) (PR interval increases with each beat and then results in an isolated P wave)

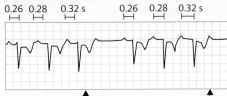
0.26 0.28   0.32 s   0.26   0.28   0.32 s

The PR interval progressively increases and then there is one isolated P wave without a following QRS complex; the PR interval then goes back to normal and starts to increase again

Third degree (complete) block (QRS complexes are independent of P waves)

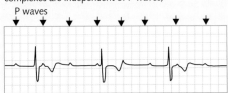
P waves

There are 90 P waves/min. There is no relationship between P waves and QRS complexes

Fig. 3.16 Classification of heart blocks. Note that only the large squares of the ECG are shown for clarity.

- Supraventricular (originating in the atrium or atrioventricular node) OR ventricular (originating in the ventricle).
- Narrow complex (describes supraventricular) OR broad complex (describes ventricular).
- Persistent OR paroxysmal (intermittent attacks).
- Heart block.

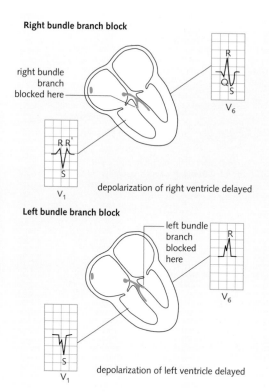

Fig. 3.17 Left and right bundle branch blocks. Disruption of the conduction system delays activation of ventricular muscle producing a characteristic split peak in the ECG.

Altered sinus rhythms

Sinus tachycardia and sinus bradycardia are produced by autonomic nervous activity and manifest as changes in rate with a regular rhythm and conduction.

Sinus tachycardia (>100 bpm in adults) usually results from:

- Exercise.
- Anxiety or excitement.
- Fever.

Sinus bradycardia (<60 bpm) commonly occurs in:

- Athletes.
- Raised intracranial pressure.
- Hypothermia

Mechanisms of arrhythmia

Broadly speaking, arrhythmias can arise as a result of any or a combination of the following:

- Interruption of the normal conduction pathway.
- Abnormal impulse generation.
- The presence of an abnormal conduction pathway.

Arrhythmias can be caused by numerous factors. These can be cardiac, such as ischaemia, structural damage, aberrant conduction pathways or mitral valve disease, or non-cardiac, such as electrolyte imbalance, drugs or caffeine.

Heart block (Fig. 3.16)

This is an interruption of the normal conduction through the atrioventricular conduction tissue. It may be classified as first-, second- or third-degree block:

- In first-degree heart block, all atrial impulses reach the ventricle, but conduction through the atrioventricular tissue takes longer than normal (P–R interval on an electrocardiogram is >0.2 s).
- In second-degree heart block, some atrial impulses fail to reach the ventricles while others succeed (not all P waves are followed by QRS complexes). Second-degree block can be divided into Mobitz type I and Mobitz type II. In type I (Wenckebach), the degree of block increases over a few beats (P–R interval increases over three or four beats, followed by an isolated P wave). This is analogous to a 'lazy' AV node which can still function. Type II is characterized by an unexpected non-conducted atrial impulse. Thus, the P–R and R–R intervals between conducted beats are constant. This is analogous to a fracture in the His–Purkinje system which is about to become completely severed. This frequently progresses to complete heart block and is associated with sudden cardiac death.
- In third-degree heart block, the atria and ventricles beat independently of each other. The ventricular rate is usually about 20–40 bpm (P waves and QRS complexes have no fixed relationship).

Bundle branch block (Fig. 3.17)

When conduction is blocked in one of the bundle branches of the interventricular septum, the affected areas of myocardium will be stimulated later by conduction from unaffected areas of myocardium. This leads to widening and disruption of the QRS complexes (>0.12 s). Looking at leads V_1 and V_6 in right bundle branch block there is:

- A second R wave (R′) in V_1 and a deeper, wider S wave in V_6.
- The last part of the QRS in lead V_1 is positive. This is because of the delayed right ventricular depolarization.

In left bundle branch block:

- There is a Q wave with an S wave in V_1.
- There is a notched R wave in V_6.
- The last part of the QRS in lead V_1 is negative. This reflects the delayed depolarization of the left ventricle.

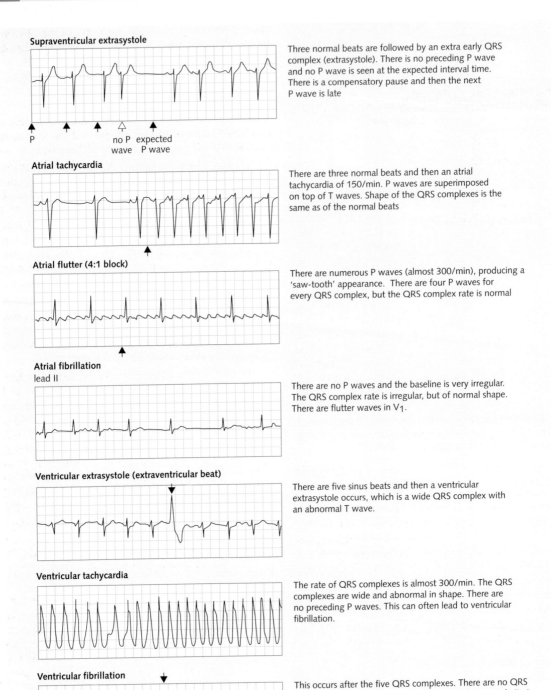

Supraventricular extrasystole

Three normal beats are followed by an extra early QRS complex (extrasystole). There is no preceding P wave and no P wave is seen at the expected interval time. There is a compensatory pause and then the next P wave is late

P   no P expected
      wave   P wave

Atrial tachycardia

There are three normal beats and then an atrial tachycardia of 150/min. P waves are superimposed on top of T waves. Shape of the QRS complexes is the same as of the normal beats

Atrial flutter (4:1 block)

There are numerous P waves (almost 300/min), producing a 'saw-tooth' appearance. There are four P waves for every QRS complex, but the QRS complex rate is normal

Atrial fibrillation
lead II

There are no P waves and the baseline is very irregular. The QRS complex rate is irregular, but of normal shape. There are flutter waves in V_1.

Ventricular extrasystole (extraventricular beat)

There are five sinus beats and then a ventricular extrasystole occurs, which is a wide QRS complex with an abnormal T wave.

Ventricular tachycardia

The rate of QRS complexes is almost 300/min. The QRS complexes are wide and abnormal in shape. There are no preceding P waves. This can often lead to ventricular fibrillation.

Ventricular fibrillation

This occurs after the five QRS complexes. There are no QRS complexes, the baseline wanders, and there is no regularity to the ECG. The ventricular wall is fibrillating and there is no organized contraction. Immediate intervention is necessary as death is imminent.

Fig. 3.18 Common atrial and ventricular arrhythmias.

HINTS AND TIPS

To determine the type of bundle branch block, look at leads V_1 and V_6 and think of WiLLiaM MaRRoW. In LBBB, there is a W pattern in lead V_1, and an M pattern in V_6 (WiLLiaM). In RBBB, there is an M pattern in lead V_1, and a W pattern in V_6 (MaRRoW).

Extrasystole (ectopic beats)

Extrasystole occurs when an abnormal beat is generated in an area of myocardium before the next sinus beat. The impulse that is generated goes on to contract the ventricle. Atrial extrasystole (narrow and irregular) or ventricular extrasystole (broad and irregular) may occur, depending upon where the impulse originates. The contraction initiated by the extrasystole is usually a weak one. This is because the reuptake of Ca^{2+} into the sarcoplasmic reticulum is not complete when contraction is stimulated so does not allow the normal degree of increase in cytosolic $[Ca^{2+}]$. Usually, there is a gap before the next normal sinus beat; it is usually this gap, or the subsequent beat (often strong due to blood pooling in the ventricle that was not ejected by the weak extrasystolic contraction and prolonged ventricular filling), that is noticed by the patient.

Wolff–Parkinson–White syndrome

The Wolff–Parkinson–White syndrome is a good example of supraventricular arrhythmia caused by the presence of an accessory (extra) conduction pathway (the bundle of Kent) between the atria and ventricles. This additional pathway can cause arrhythmia by causing pre-excitation and/or a phenomenon called re-entry. The additional pathway conducts faster than the AV node and certain areas of ventricular myocardium will be excited before others; this is pre-excitation. Re-entry occurs when depolarization of ventricular myocardium is propagated retrogradely via the additional pathway and re-excites the atria.

Supraventricular tachycardias

Atrial tachycardia and atrial flutter are caused by an abnormal focus in the atrium or an abnormal conduction pathway causing re-entry that results in atrial contraction at a rapid rate.

In atrial flutter the rate is usually around 300 bpm but not all atrial impulses are conducted to the ventricle. Often, the ratio of atrial to ventricular beats is 2:1 or 3:1.

These are usually characterized by a regular rhythm at a rate between 140 and 220 bpm, with narrow QRS complexes.

Atrial fibrillation

Atrial fibrillation (AF) is a common arrhythmia and a significant cause of morbidity, particularly in elderly people, occurring in around 10% of those over 75. In AF, electrical activity in the atria is chaotic and depolarization occurs at a rate of 300–600 bpm. This does not produce effective atrial contraction, merely a rippling effect in the muscle (fibrillation). Ventricular activity is also affected because impulses are sporadically conducted through the AV node allowing variable time for ventricular filling between beats, producing a characteristic 'irregularly irregular' pulse in rate and volume. AF can be persistent, permanent or paroxysmal.

This chaotic activity is due to:

- The presence of numerous ectopic foci for impulse generation.
- The presence of numerous re-entry circuits that become repeatedly excited within the atria.

It is commonly caused by mitral valve disease, ischaemic heart disease, thyrotoxicosis, hypertension and excessive alcohol consumption. The lack of effective atrial contraction and resulting stasis of blood predisposes to the development of a thrombus (blood clot) within the left atrium, which can throw off emboli that can pass to the brain causing ischaemic stroke, or to other visceral organs causing ischaemia or infarction. AF is the most important cause of stroke in elderly patients and must not be ignored. Some patients with AF will suffer from palpitation or may experience dizziness or syncope (fainting).

There are two approaches to treating atrial fibrillation and there is ongoing debate as to which is superior. These are:

- Rate control: aims to reduce the ventricular rate. Drugs used to control the rate include Ca^{2+} channel blockers (e.g. verapamil), beta-blockers and digoxin.
- Rhythm control: aims to restore sinus rhythm. This can be achieved electrically by DC cardioversion or pharmacologically with drugs such as flecainide (Na^+ channel blocker) or amiodarone.

Currently it appears that if patients are asymptomatic then rate control is better than rhythm control. If sinus rhythm cannot be restored, people with chronic AF should be considered for anticoagulation with warfarin to reduce the risk of embolic events such as stroke. The CHADS2 score predicts the risk of stroke and thus is useful when deciding whether or not to anticoagulate these patients (Fig. 3.19).

Fig. 3.19 The CHADS2 score*

Factor	Score
Congestive cardiac failure	1
Hypertension	1
Age >75	1
Diabetes mellitus	1
Stroke or TIA	2

0 = low risk ⟶ aspirin
1 = moderate risk ⟶ warfarin
2+ = high risk ⟶ warfarin

The CHADS2 score is used as a guide when making decisions about anticoagulation in patients with atrial fibrillation (AF). It applies to patients in persistent and paroxysmal AF (TIA, transient is chaemic attack).

Ventricular arrhythmias

Ventricular tachycardia

Ventricular tachycardia occurs when impulses originate from an ectopic focus or a re-entry circuit within the ventricles. It is characterized by broad QRS complexes (i.e. duration >100 ms) on an ECG at a rate of >120 bpm.

Ventricular fibrillation

An irregular, uncoordinated, rippling contraction of the ventricles. There is no effective cardiac output, leading to rapid loss of consciousness, as perfusion of the brain is interrupted. Death results unless effective treatment is initiated immediately. This often occurs secondary to myocardial infarction and is thought to be the underlying arrhythmia in the majority of cases of sudden cardiac death.

Cardiac arrest

Cardiac arrest occurs when there is an absence of cardiac output. Basic life support should be commenced immediately while the cardiac arrest team is called, and a cardiac monitor attached to the patient. There are two main types of cardiac arrest: 'shockable' and 'non-shockable', referring to whether or not they respond to defibrillation.
'Shockable' rhythms include:

- Ventricular fibrillation.
- Ventricular tachycardia.

'Non-shockable' rhythms include:

- Pulseless electrical activity: the electrical activity of the heart is compatible with an output but there is no pulse.
- Asystole: an absence of cardiac electrical activity.

Once the type of cardiac arrest has been determined a strict algorithm is followed, as outlined in Fig. 3.20.

Cardiac arrest into a 'shockable' rhythm is usually due to a cardiac cause. Defibrillation attempts to stop the abnormal electrical activity in the hope that the SA node will regain control.

Cardiac arrest into a 'non-shockable' rhythm is usually from a non-cardiac cause. These are divided into four 'H's and four 'T's:

- Hypovolaemia.
- Hypothermia.
- Hypotension.
- Hypo/hyperkalaemia and metabolic disturbances.
- Tension pneumothorax.
- Tamponade (pericardial).
- Thromboembolic.
- Toxic and therapeutic.

Cardiac arrests occur regularly in the hospital setting, although in a number of situations a 'Do Not attempt Resuscitation' or 'DNR' order is put in place. These are written by senior members of staff when it is thought that death is expected, resuscitation under the circumstances would be futile, or the patient's quality of life subsequently would be very poor. These are obviously very difficult decisions to make, and a sound knowledge of ethical principles and medical law is essential.

Anti-arrhythmic drugs

The aims of drug treatment include:

- To decrease myocyte excitability.
- To increase the refractory period.
- To slow conduction.

The Vaughan Williams classification system is used for anti-arrhythmic drugs and is based on their actions.

Class I: sodium channel blockers

These drugs can be subdivided into class IA (e.g. quinidine, procainamide), class IB (e.g. lidocaine, tocainide) and class IC (e.g. flecainide). They all act by blocking fast voltage-gated Na^+ channels and are said to have a membrane stabilizing effect such that they increase the threshold for depolarization and slow the upstroke of the action potential. They also prolong the absolute refractory period.

Class II: beta-blockers

Class II drugs (e.g. propranolol and atenolol) block the increase in pacemaker activity and increase the speed of conduction that is produced by sympathetic stimulation of β adrenoceptors.

Beta-blockers may be used for ectopic beats, atrial fibrillation and atrial tachycardia. They are indicated when circulating catecholamines are too high (e.g. after a myocardial infarction and in thyrotoxicosis).

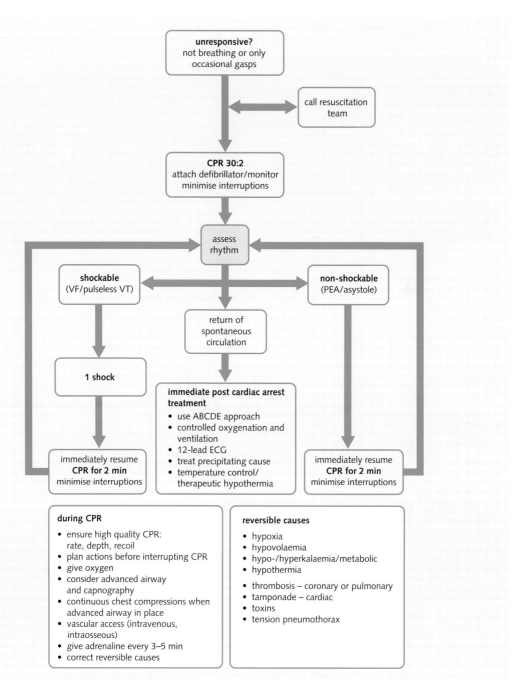

Fig. 3.20 Cardiac arrest algorithm. (Reproduced with the kind permission of the Resuscitation Council (UK).

Class III: potassium channel blockers

Class III drugs (e.g. amiodarone) block K^+ channels, slowing repolarization (phase 3), leading to a prolonged action potential and refractory period. Side-effects of amiodarone are important, common, and affect multiple organs. These include interstitial lung disease, hypo- or hyperthyroidism and deranged liver function to name a few.

Class IV: calcium channel blockers

Class IV drugs (e.g. verapamil) block L-type Ca^{2+} channels, thereby decreasing the gradient of the pacemaker potential, slowing the rate of depolarization in the SA node and prolonging the conduction delay in the AV node. They also have negative inotropic effects by limiting the influx of Ca^{2+} during the plateau phase.

Other drugs not in this classification

- Digoxin: has a central effect, stimulating the vagus nerve and increasing parasympathetic stimulation, thus slowing the heart rate. It simultaneously exerts its positive inotropic effect by inhibition of the Na^+/K^+ATPase.
- Adenosine: causes hyperpolarization at the AV node by increasing K^+ permeability. This causes a transient complete heart block at the AV node. It can be used diagnostically to unmask surpaventricular arrhythmias or to terminate them.

Drugs used to treat bradyarrythmias

Drugs that can be used in the treatment of bradyarrhythmias include:

- Anticholinergics (e.g. atropine): antagonize the parasympathetic effects on the SA node and AV node, increasing heart rate.
- Sympathomimetics (e.g. isoprenaline): stimulate the β_1 receptors in the SA node and AV node, increasing heart rate.

These drugs are useful in the acute setting but are of limited benefit long term. Atropine causes side-effects including dry mouth and constipation, and isoprenaline must be given intravenously, making it impractical.

Other treatments for arrhythmias

Carotid sinus massage

Massaging the carotid sinuses in the neck causes a baroreceptor-mediated increase in parasympathetic activity (explained in Ch. 6) that slows the firing rate of the SA node and prolongs delay at the AV node. This approach can terminate some supraventricular tachycardias.

Direct current (DC) shock therapy

Cardioversion is performed to return the heart to sinus rhythm. This can be achieved using an electrical current (DC cardioversion) or pharmacologically. Defibrillation, as the name suggests, is the use of an electric current to terminate ventricular fibrillation.

Cardioversion can be used in a number of arrhythmias including AF, atrial flutter and fast ventricular tachycardia to restore normal sinus rhythm. In DC cardioversion, the shock must be synchronized with the R wave on the ECG. This ensures that the shock is not delivered during the relative refractory period, and thus alleviates the risk of inducing ventricular fibrillation.

Implantable cardiac defibrillators (ICD) are available and can be implanted into patients. These ICD devices detect ventricular arrhythmias and act either by delivering a small shock to return the heart to sinus rhythm or by overdrive pacing, whereby the ventricle is paced rapidly out of the arrhythmia and then slowed back down to a normal rate.

Radiofrequency ablation

In this procedure, a catheter is passed up into the heart via the femoral vein, and radiofrequency energy is used to produce a lesion in the myocardium. It can be used to 'ablate' focuses of ectopic activity or to interrupt aberrant conduction pathways. It is used primarily in the treatment of supraventricular arrhythmias including atrial fibrillation. Many of the ectopic foci that underlie AF in structurally normal hearts originate in the roots of the pulmonary veins. By ablating the myocardium between the pulmonary veins and the atria, conduction between the two is interrupted. This technique, called pulmonary vein isolation, can abolish AF in many cases, and its use is on the increase.

Pacemaker

Pacemaker implantation is the principal treatment for bradycardia and allows the heart rate to be controlled. Pacemakers are used in sick sinus syndrome where there is disease of the sinus node (ischaemia, infarction or degeneration) leading to pauses in sinus node function and bradycardia. They are also used for complete heart block and Mobitz type II block (as this frequently progresses to complete heart block). The most widely used pacemakers are dual chamber pacemakers, which have an electrode in the right atrium and the right ventricle. This allows independent control of the atria and the ventricles, which can be manipulated to optimize cardiac function.

The cardiac cycle and control of cardiac output

4

● Objectives

You should be able to:

- Describe the stages of the ventricular cycle and the pressure/volume changes that take place.
- Describe the stages of the atrial cycle and the corresponding changes in the jugular venous pressure.
- Describe the normal and added heart sounds.
- Understand what a murmur is and why they occur.
- Describe the common causes, haemodynamic changes, symptoms and signs of common valvular abnormalities.
- Understand the principles and common indications for echocardiography.
- Understand the definition and significance of preload, afterload and contractility.
- Understand the physiological and pharmacological factors that affect contractility.
- Describe Starling's law of the heart and its implications.

THE CARDIAC CYCLE

The cardiac cycle is the sequence of pressure and volume changes that take place during cardiac activity (Figs 4.1 and 4.2). At a resting heart rate of approximately 70 beats per minute (bpm), the cardiac cycle lasts 0.85 seconds. This is divided into diastole, which lasts 0.6 s and systole, which lasts 0.25 s. When considering the cardiac cycle, it is useful to remember that:

- Blood flows down a pressure gradient.
- The state of a valve is dependent on the pressure gradient across it.

The ventricular cycle

The ventricular cycle consists of four phases. The duration and order of each of these phases is shown in Fig. 4.2.

1. Ventricular filling (diastole)

The atria and ventricles are all relaxed initially, and there is passive filling of the atria and ventricles as a result of central venous pressure and pulmonary venous pressure (right and left side respectively). The volume increases until a neutral ventricular volume is reached. Further filling makes the ventricle distend, causing ventricular pressure to rise. This passive ventricular filling will stop when ventricular pressure reaches central venous/pulmonary venous pressure. Contraction of the atria further increases the filling of the ventricles. This accounts for only about 15–20% of ventricular filling at rest. During exercise, however, when heart rate is increased, the atrial contraction becomes more important

as the time for passive ventricular filling is reduced. The volume of blood in the ventricle at the end of diastole is termed the end-diastolic volume (EDV).

HINTS AND TIPS

This 'atrial kick' is absent in people with atrial fibrillation due to the ineffective atrial contraction. This has little effect on cardiac output at rest.

2. Isovolumetric contraction (systole)

Contraction of the ventricles increases ventricular pressure. Ventricular pressure rises above atrial pressure, closing the atrioventricular valves early in systole. This creates a closed chamber as all valves are closed. As ventricular contraction proceeds, wall tension increases, causing a rapid rise in ventricular pressure. The rate of rise in pressure is a measure of cardiac contractility. During this isovolumetric phase, no blood is ejected from the ventricles because aortic/pulmonary pressure is greater than that in the ventricles, maintaining the aortic and pulmonary valves in their closed position.

3. Ejection (systole)

As contraction proceeds, ventricular pressure eventually rises above arterial pressure, opening the arterial (aortic and pulmonary) valves. This causes rapid ejection of blood from the ventricles and a rapid initial rise in arterial pressure. The momentum of blood prevents immediate valve closure, even when ventricular pressure falls below arterial pressure. Eventually, the

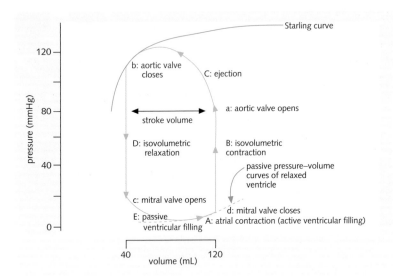

Fig. 4.1 Pressure–volume cycle of left ventricle. The most significant pressure changes occur within the ventricles during the isovolumetric stages.

Fig. 4.2 Summary table of the stages of the cardiac cycle

	Diastole	Systole		Diastole
Stage	Ventricular filling	Isovolumetric contraction	Ejection	Isovolumetric relaxation
Duration (s)	0.5	0.05	0.3	0.08
AV valves	Open	Closed	Closed	Closed
Arterial valves	Closed	Closed	Open	Closed
Ventricular pressure	Falls then slowly rises	Rapid rise	Rises then slowly falls	Rapid fall
Ventricular volume	Increases	Constant	Decreases	Constant

Note: changes at fixed volume are referred to as isovolumetric, and precede the later contraction or dilation of the ventricles (AV, atrioventricular).

arterial valves close, creating a brief rise in arterial pressure called the dicrotic notch. It is important to note that the ventricle does not empty completely. There is an end-systolic volume of about 40–50%, which can be used to increase stroke volume when necessary. The proportion of end-diastolic volume ejected during systole is referred to as the ejection fraction, and is usually between 50%–60%.

HINTS AND TIPS

Venous return = Right heart input & output = Pulmonary blood flow = Left heart input & output = Systemic blood flow. This is because they are all in series, and this idea that what goes in must come out is called the Fick principle.

4. Isovolumetric relaxation (diastole)

Again, both sets of valves are closed as the ventricles relax creating an enclosed chamber. When ventricular pressure falls below atrial pressure, the atrioventricular valves open and the cycle repeats.

The atrial cycle

The pressure changes in the atria during the cardiac cycle are different from those in the ventricles. The right atrium directly communicates with the internal jugular veins (IJV) and the absence of valves between the two means that changes in right atrial pressure are reflected by changes in the jugular venous pressure (JVP). The JVP waveform is assessed when examining the cardiovascular system and is shown in Fig. 4.3. The JVP waveform has five components:

- The A wave is caused by atrial contraction. Although the tricuspid valve is open, this still causes transient backpressure into the vena cava and IJV.
- The C wave coincides with closure of the tricuspid valve.
- The X descent occurs after the C wave as the atria relax, decreasing pressure.
- The V wave occurs during systole as a result of atrial filling. As atrial pressure rises against a closed valve, it creates backpressure, giving rise to the V wave.
- The Y descent occurs due to passive ventricular filling during diastole.

Heart sounds

Normal heart sounds (Fig. 4.4)

- First (S1): produced by closure of the mitral and tricuspid valves.
- Second (S2): produced by closure of the aortic and pulmonary valves.

Splitting of the second heart sound (Fig. 4.5)

During inspiration, physiological splitting of the second heart sound can occur. Inspiration decreases intrathoracic pressure, increasing venous return and right ventricular preload. Simultaneously, the lungs expand, decreasing

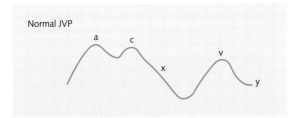

Fig. 4.3 The normal jugular venous pressure (JVP) waveform (a, a wave; c, c wave; v, v wave; x, x descent; y, y descent).

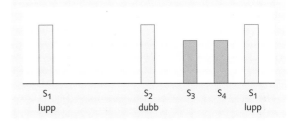

Fig. 4.4 Normal heart sounds (S_1, first heart sound; S_2, second heart sound) and the added third and fourth heart sounds (S_3, third heart sound; S_4, fourth heart sound).

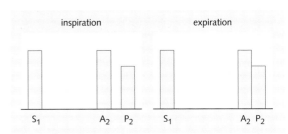

Fig. 4.5 Splitting of the second heart sound. S_2 may show physiological splitting into A_2 and P_2 (A_2, aortic component; P_2, pulmonary component).

return to the left atrium and decreasing left ventricular preload. As a result, right ventricular systole lasts longer than left ventricular systole and the pulmonary valve closes after the aortic valve. This difference can be heard as splitting of S2.

Added heart sounds (Fig. 4.4)

- Third (S3): can be heard in early diastole and is caused by rapid ventricular filling. A third heart sound is common in young people and athletes. It may also be present in people with heart failure.
- Fourth (S4): occurs just before the first heart sound and is due to forceful atrial contraction against a stiff ventricle. This is always abnormal and can occur in the presence of ventricular hypertrophy, which makes the ventricle less compliant.

Fig. 4.6 brings together the atrial cycle, ventricular cycle and heart sounds, showing their temporal relation to each other.

HINTS AND TIPS

To get an idea of the timing of the third and fourth heart sounds, consider the cadence of the words Tennessee (mirrors the third heart sound) and Kentucky (mirrors the fourth heart sound).

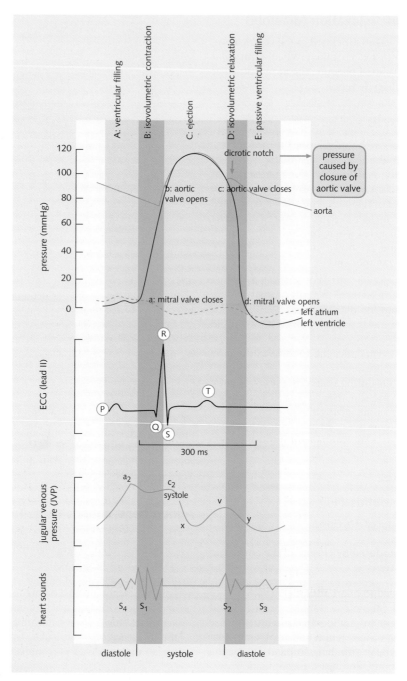

Fig. 4.6 Displayed at the top of the diagram are the pressures in the left atrium, left ventricle and aorta during the cardiac cycle. Pressure in the left ventricle increases slightly during left atrial contraction (A). The most rapid increase in pressure occurs during isovolumetric contraction (B). The increase in pressure caused by ventricular contraction closes the mitral valve (a). When left ventricular pressure just exceeds aortic pressure the aortic valve opens (b) leading to ejection (C). Pressure rises to a peak and then falls, leading to aortic valve closure (c). Isovolumetric relaxation then occurs (D) and eventually left ventricular pressure is just below left atrial pressure, leading to the opening of the mitral valve (d). This allows passive filling of the ventricles (E). Below this the normal electrocardiogram is displayed as it relates to the cardiac cycle. The jugular venous pressure (JVP) (shown below) reflects right atrial pressure due to the close proximity of the central veins to the right atrium. Finally, the heart sounds are displayed (S_1, closure of the mitral and tricuspid valves 'lubb'; S_2, closure of the aortic and pulmonary valves 'dupp').

Murmurs

Murmurs can be heard with a stethoscope and result from the presence of turbulent blood flow. Although most often due to valvular disease, this is not always the case. A benign (harmless) murmur may be present in young people or people in high cardiac output states such as pregnancy or anaemia. Murmurs may also be present in congenital heart defects such as septal defects or patent ductus arteriosus. When describing murmurs, you should consider when in the cardiac cycle it occurs (systolic or diastolic), the nature of the murmur and where it is heard loudest.

> If flow is very turbulent, loud murmurs can sometimes be felt with the hand on the chest wall. This is called a thrill.

> **HINTS AND TIPS**
>
> The volume of a murmur does not indicate the severity of valvular heart disease!

VALVULAR HEART DISEASE

Valvular disease can manifest as either stenosis or regurgitation, or sometimes both simultaneously. Stenosis is an obstruction to normal flow through the valve and can be likened to a narrowing of the valve. Regurgitation is when the valve fails in its function to prevent backflow of blood, analogous to a leaky valve. This can also be described as an incompetent valve or insufficient valve.

Valvular disease can be caused by:

- Direct damage to the valve leaflets (usually the case in stenosis).
- Damage to the valve ring (the annulus).
- Damage to the supporting structures (papillary muscles, chordae tendinae).

The most commonly affected valves are the aortic and mitral valves. This is due to the high pressures to which they are exposed (compared to those in the right side). The clinical features and findings on examination of the common valve pathologies are shown in Fig. 4.7.

Mitral stenosis

Mitral stenosis occurs most commonly as a result of rheumatic heart disease. The stenosis limits passive filling of the left ventricle during diastole, increasing the contribution of atrial systole. It also causes an increase in left atrial pressure, causing distension of the atrium (often causing atrial fibrillation) and increasing pulmonary venous pressure.

Mitral regurgitation

Mitral regurgitation can result from infective endocarditis, ischaemic damage to the chordae tendinae or papillary muscles, or ventricular dilatation. The volume of blood that flows back into the left atrium during systole causes dilatation of the atrium (often causing atrial fibrillation) and increases pulmonary venous pressures, which can lead to pulmonary oedema. With time, the left ventricle also becomes dilated.

Aortic stenosis

Aortic stenosis usually occurs as a result of calcification of a normal aortic valve or congenitally bicuspid aortic valve (tends to occur at a younger age). It can also result from rheumatic heart disease. The stenosed valve increases the afterload on the left ventricle, increasing the force required to eject blood into the aorta. This causes hypertrophy of the left ventricle. The reduction in cardiac output can result in breathlessness and inadequate perfusion of tissues such as the brain (causing syncope). Reduced myocardial perfusion combined with the increased myocardial oxygen demand can also cause angina.

Aortic regurgitation

Aortic regurgitation can result from infective endocarditis, dilatation of the aortic root (e.g. in Marfan's syndrome) or rheumatic heart disease. The backflow of blood into the left ventricle causes ventricular dilatation and in order to maintain cardiac output, left ventricular hypertrophy occurs. If onset is acute, these compensatory structural changes cannot take place and the increase in left ventricular pressure causes premature closure of the mitral valve and prevents diastolic filling.

Echocardiography

Echocardiography is commonly used in the diagnosis and assessment of valvular heart disease. The procedure uses an ultrasound probe, which is placed on the anterior chest wall (transthoracic echocardiography, TTE). Ultrasonic waves generated by the probe are reflected back at tissue interfaces and picked up by the probe. Echoes from tissues furthest from the transmitter take longest to return and different tissues reflect waves differently, allowing an image to be built up. Traditionally, echocardiography produces a 2D image but 3D imaging is becoming increasingly available.

Advantages of echocardiography for cardiovascular investigation include:

- Non-invasive, painless, and harmless.
- Can be used to study the motion of the heart and valves.
- Can be used to measure velocity of blood (using the Doppler shift phenomenon) and to estimate

Fig. 4.7 Causes, symptoms and signs in common valvular abnormalities

	Common causes	Symptoms	Signs
Aortic stenosis	Calcification of a normal or bicuspid valve	Syncope Angina Dyspnoea	Slow rising pulse Quiet S_2 Ejection systolic murmur radiating to neck 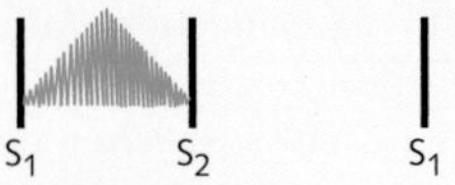 S_1 S_2 S_1 Heaving apex beat
Aortic regurgitation	Aortic dilatation Endocarditis	Breathlessness (occurs with the development of heart failure)	Collapsing pulse Early diastolic murmur 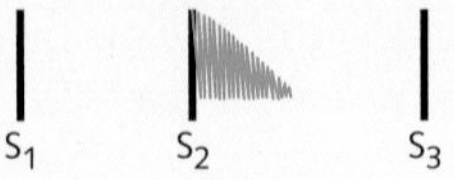 S_1 S_2 S_3
Mitral stenosis	Rheumatic fever	Exertional breathlessness Fatigue Palpitation (due to AF)	Malar flush Loud S_1 Mid diastolic murmur 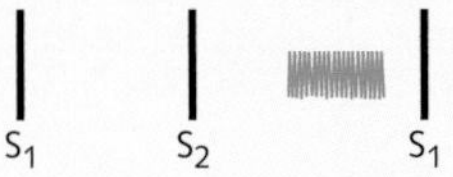 S_1 S_2 S_1
Mitral regurgitation	Ventricular dilatation MI Endocarditis Valve prolapse	Exertional dyspnoea Palpitation (due to AF)	Pansystolic murmur radiating to the axilla 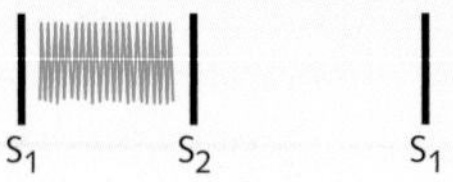 S_1 S_2 S_1

stenosis severity from acceleration of blood through a valve.

- Can be used to assess left ventricular size and function in the assessment of heart failure.
- Can be used to assess the aortic root and pericardial effusions.

Disadvantages include the fact that the ribs and lungs (due to the volume of air) do not allow ultrasound waves to pass through them, so special sites (or windows) must be used. Most imaging is still done through the anterior chest wall, but, when necessary, an oesophageal probe can be used to perform transoesophageal echocardiography (TOE). Examples of images of TTE and TOE images are shown in Figs 4.8 and 4.9 respectively.

Rheumatic heart disease

Rheumatic heart disease is a consequence of rheumatic fever that may have occurred many years previously. The acute process can leave the valves scarred and deformed, causing chronic rheumatic heart disease.

Acute rheumatic fever is an inflammatory disease caused by an autoimmune reaction initiated by infection with group A streptococci, usually in the throat. It usually affects children aged 5–15 years but is now rare in the UK because of improved sanitation and the use of antibiotics to effectively treat streptococcal infections. It affects the heart, skin, joints, and central nervous system. The Duckett Jones criteria for diagnosis include:

- Carditis involving all three layers (pancarditis).
- Sydenham's chorea (St Vitus dance; rapid, involuntary purposeless movements).
- Polyarthritis affecting the large joints.
- Erythema marginatum (macular rash with erythematous edge).
- Subcutaneous nodules.

Fever, arthralgia and leukocytosis also commonly occur.

Carditis consists of granulomatous lesions with a central necrotic area (Aschoff nodule), initially with an inflammatory infiltrate that is eventually replaced by fibrous tissue. Commonly, it affects the mitral valve

A

B

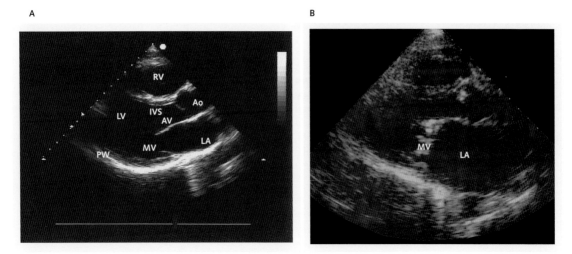

Fig. 4.8 (A) Normal echocardiogram of the parasternal long axis view (diastolic frame) (Ao, aorta; AV, aortic valve; IVS, intraventricular septum; LA, left atrium; LV, left ventricle; MV, mitral valve; PW, posterior LV wall; RV, right ventricle). (B) Echocardiogram of mitral stenosis (long axis). The mitral valve (MV) leaflets are densely thickened and the left atrium (LA) is severely dilated. (Courtesy of Dr A Timmis and Dr S Brecker.)

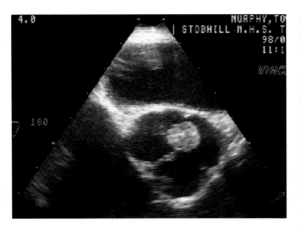

Fig. 4.9 Transoesophageal echocardiography (TOE) image.

(65%) or the mitral and aortic valves (25%). In the long term it can lead to commissural fusion (fusing of valve leaflets), shortening/thickening of the chordae and cusp fibrosis – the so-called fish-mouth or button-hole mitral valve deformity. This can result in stenosis or regurgitation of the mitral or aortic valves.

Infective endocarditis

Infective endocarditis is an infection of the endocardium, usually involving the heart valves. Previously, endocarditis was classified as acute or subacute; now it is

classified according to the causative organism. The incidence is 6–7 per 100 000 in the UK, but it is more common in developing countries.

Infective endocarditis occurs more commonly on valves that have been previously damaged or are congenitally abnormal. Inflammation of the valve causes destruction and scarring. Vegetations (consisting of fibrin, platelets and the infecting organism) usually develop on the valves causing damage and often, valvular regurgitation. These vegetations can also throw off emboli to other organs such as the kidneys and brain causing ischaemia. Until proven otherwise, any patient with a fever and a new murmur should be investigated and potentially treated for endocarditis. The main aim of treatment is to resolve the infection using intravenous (IV) antibiotics but multiple sets of blood cultures from multiple sites should be taken before starting antibiotics to increase the chance of identifying the causative organism. Any acute valvular abnormalities (if severe) may need to be treated surgically. The common causative organisms include:

- *Streptococcus viridans*: subacute; common after dental procedures, tonsillectomy or bronchoscopy.
- *Staphylococcus aureus*: acute; common in patients with indwelling catheters and in IV drug users.
- *Enterococcus faecalis*: common in patients with pelvic infections or after having pelvic surgery.
- *Coxiella burnetii* (Q fever): subacute.
- *Staphylococcus epidermidis, Aspergillus, Candida, Brucella, Histoplasma*: more common in IV drug users and in patients with prosthetic heart valves.

CONTROL OF CARDIAC OUTPUT

Definitions and concepts

Cardiac output (CO) is the amount of blood ejected from the heart in 1 minute. It is a product of the stroke volume (SV) and heart rate (HR) (CO = SV × HR). In a normal adult, it ranges from 4 to 7 L/min at rest but is increased during exercise (up to 20 L/min) and decreased during sleep, in line with the body's metabolic requirements. Before considering how cardiac output is regulated, it is important to understand a number of definitions:

- Stroke volume (SV): the volume of blood ejected in one ventricular contraction.
- Stroke work (SW): the amount of external energy expended in one ventricular contraction. SW is the mean arterial blood pressure (MABP) multiplied by the SV.
- Contractility: the force of contraction for a given fibre length.
- End-diastolic volume (EDV): the volume of blood in the ventricle just before contraction.
- End-diastolic pressure (EDP): the pressure of blood in the ventricle just before contraction.
- End-systolic volume (ESV): the volume of blood left in the ventricle after contraction.
- Central venous pressure (CVP): the pressure of blood in the great veins as they enter the right atrium.
- Venous return (VR): the volume of blood returning to the right heart in 1 minute. In a healthy heart VR = CO.
- Total peripheral resistance (TPR): the resistance to the flow of blood in the whole system (MABP/CO).
- Systemic vascular resistance (SVR): the resistance to blood flow offered by all of the systemic vasculature (this excludes the pulmonary vasculature). It is calculated as (MABP − CVP)/CO.
- Ejection fraction: the proportion of EDV that is ejected during systole.

> Stroke volume, and therefore cardiac output, is influenced by three factors:
> - Preload.
> - Afterload.
> - Contractility.

Preload

Preload is defined as the degree of ventricular myocyte stretch at the end of diastole and is determined by the EDV. The greater the EDV, the greater the preload and vice versa. EDV is influenced by:

- Venous return: influenced by blood volume, venous tone, gravity, respiration, skeletal muscle contraction (for more detail see Ch. 5)

- Heart rate: at high heart rates, the duration of diastole and thus time for passive ventricular filling is reduced, decreasing EDV.
- Atrial contraction: ineffective atrial contraction, as occurs in atrial fibrillation, will reduce EDV.

> Some people will think of preload in terms of end–diastolic pressure and others in term of end-diastolic volume. It is the EDV that determines the fibre length at the onset of contraction and therefore the strength of contraction but when ventricular compliance is normal, end-diastolic pressure is just as accurate. The distinction is important only when ventricular compliance is altered.

Afterload

Afterload is defined as the force or stress on myocytes during systole. Think of it as the force against which the ventricle has to contract. It is determined by the resistance to outflow from the ventricle. For the left ventricle, aortic pressure is the main determinant and for the right ventricle, pulmonary artery pressure is the main determinant. Afterload is also increased by valvular stenosis.

Contractility

As described in Chapter 3, contractility is the force of contraction for a given fibre length and is determined by the degree of Ca^{2+} influx during the plateau phase (phase 3) of the cardiac action potential. Factors that affect contractility are termed inotropic factors. Examples of positive and negative inotropes include:

Positive inotropes

- Catecholamines: noradrenaline/norepinephrine released by sympathetic nerves and circulating adrenaline/epinephrine and noradrenaline/norepinephrine bind β_1 receptors on cardiac myocytes. The resulting increase in levels of cAMP opens L-type Ca^{2+} channels, increasing Ca^{2+} entry into the cytosol during the plateau phase of the action potential. Catecholamines also increase the activity of the sarcoplasmic reticulum (SR) Ca^{2+}ATPase, increasing reuptake of Ca^{2+} into the SR and thus increasing the amount available for Ca^{2+} induced Ca^{2+} release during the next action potential.
- Beta-agonists (e.g. dobutamine): by the mechanisms described above.
- Phosphodiesterase inhibitors (e.g. milrinone): these drugs inhibit the breakdown of cAMP and increase opening of L-type Ca^{2+} channels.
- Ca^{2+} sensitizers (e.g. levosimendan): these drugs increase the sensitivity of the contractile proteins to

Ca^{2+}, increasing the strength of contraction for a given rise in cytosolic $[Ca^{2+}]$.

- Cardiac glycosides: digoxin is an inhibitor of the Na^+/K^+ ATPase and exerts a positive inotropic influence. By inhibiting the Na^+/K^+ ATPase, the $[Na^+]$ inside the myocyte will increase reducing the gradient for Ca^{2+} removal by the Na^+/Ca^{2+} exchanger, increasing cytosolic $[Ca^{2+}]$.

Negative inotropes

- Beta-blockers (e.g. propranolol): inhibit the action of catecholamines on β_1 receptors.
- Ca^{2+} channel blockers (e.g. verapamil): block the L-type Ca^{2+} channels on ventricular myocytes, reducing Ca^{2+} influx.
- Hypoxia.

> Although sympathetic stimulation causes an increase in contractility, parasympathetic stimulation does NOT decrease contractility because parasympathetic innervation to the ventricular myocardium is sparse.

Starling's law of the heart

'The energy released during contraction depends upon the initial fibre length' (Fig. 4.10). The greater the heart is stretched by filling (preload), then the greater the energy released by contraction. This phenomenon is due to the stretch-dependent sensitivity of myocardial contractile proteins to Ca^{2+}, which influences the number of actin–myosin cross-bridges formed, and it is known as Starling's law. It is important to distinguish this from contractility, which is the force of contraction for a given fibre length and is determined by the degree to which cytosolic $[Ca^{2+}]$ is increased.

Although the initial stretch of the ventricular myocardium, the preload, is produced by the EDV, end-diastolic pressure (EDP) is easier to measure, and the relationship between the two is almost linear (providing myocardial compliance is normal). In the right ventricle EDP is closely related to the central venous pressure (CVP). EDP plotted against SV produces the Starling curve (Fig. 4.11). Excessively high filling pressures will cause excessive myocyte stretch and the relationship is no longer valid such that when a certain EDP is exceeded, any further increase will decrease SV.

In a closed system such as the heart in which the chambers are arranged in series, what goes in must come out. This Fick principle has been mentioned previously but is very important to remember. Starling's law is the principle that matches right and left

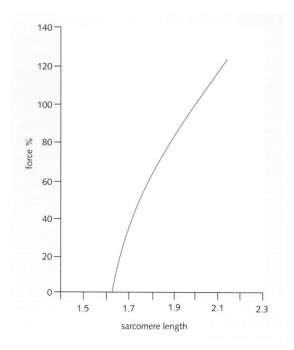

Fig. 4.10 Sarcomere length compared with tension. Increasing the initial sarcomere length increases tension, up to the maximum stretch possible for an individual myocyte.

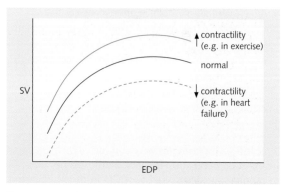

Fig. 4.11 Stroke volume (SV) compared with end-diastolic pressure (EDP). This produces the Starling curve, which shows that an increase in EDP (and therefore end-diastolic volume (EDV) as they have an almost linear relationship) causes an increased SV. There is, however, a limit at which the curve turns downwards and the relationship is no longer valid. The mechanism for this downturn is complex, and it mainly reflects excessive stretching of the ventricular myocytes. Changes in contractility are characterized by upward (positively inotropic) and downward (negatively inotropic) displacement of the Starling curve.

ventricular stroke volumes and understanding it is central to understanding how cardiac output is controlled. We will now consider how this balance is maintained in the following situations assuming constant heart rate and contractility.

Change in preload

An increase in preload, which is primarily determined by venous return, will lead to an increase in cardiac output according to Starling's law. The increased right ventricular EDV (preload) increases the initial stretch of the right ventricular myocardium. Within a few beats, the increased force of contraction and increased right ventricular SV will increase pulmonary pressures and thus increase filling of the left ventricle and left ventricular EDV. This will increase left ventricular SV (and therefore CO). Although the increase in SV is not instant, the imbalance between VR and SV is only transient. A decrease in preload will decrease CO according to the same principle.

Change in afterload

An increase in afterload will reduce the amount of blood ejected from the left ventricle, initially decreasing SV and increasing ESV. Assuming constant filling pressures, this will result in a greater EDV during the next cycle. The increased preload will increase the force of the next contraction to restore stroke volume despite the increased afterload.

> To illustrate the importance of precisely matching right and left ventricular stroke volume, consider the consequence of right SV being slightly greater than left SV. Although not a problem if transient, if such an imbalance persists, pulmonary blood volume and, as a result, pulmonary blood pressure would increase, leading to congestion and pulmonary oedema. This can occur in left ventricular heart failure.

Starling's experiments were conducted on an isolated heart–lung preparation in 1914. While it is not possible to monitor the determinants of CO in the way Starling could by isolating the heart and lungs, cardiologists can insert a single catheter from the femoral artery back up the aorta and into the left ventricle by passing it retrogradely through the aortic valve. The catheter contains conductance sensors to measure left ventricular volume and a pressure sensor at the tip. This freely records pressure–volume loops. Fig. 4.12 shows the pressure–volume loop for the left ventricle and how this is affected by changes in EDV and contractility.

Starling's findings in the controlled situation of the isolated heart–lung preparation are important in enabling clinicians to understand the importance of:

- Adequate, but not excessive filling of the ventricles (e.g. in heart failure, high EDV may be pathological).
- Keeping peripheral resistance as low as possible to maximize CO (reducing afterload).

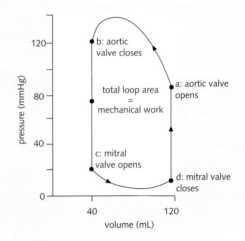

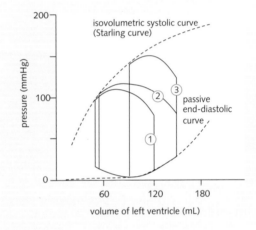

Fig. 4.12 Pressure–volume loops (1, normal state; 2, increased end-diastolic volume (EDV) leads to increased stroke volume (SV) if arterial pressure is constant; 3, increased EDV and increased MAP result in a decreased SV). The end-systolic points of the loops produce the Starling curve so long as the contractility remains constant.

- Maintaining a sufficient level of contractility to maintain life when the previous determinants have been optimized.

These factors are particularly important when considering the treatment of patients with heart failure and will be discussed further in Chapter 8.

HINTS AND TIPS

Remember that cardiac output is limited by venous return – without integrated regulation of the cardiovascular system, an increased heart rate will be compensated by reduced stroke volume.

Haemodynamics and vascular function (5)

● Objectives

You should be able to:
- Understand the principles of blood flow, viscosity and resistance.
- Describe Poiseuille's law.
- Describe the normal arterial waveform and its variations.
- Explain the basis for the changes in vascular resistance through the vascular tree, and how these changes affect blood pressure and the velocity of blood flow.
- Measure blood pressure manually and interpret Korotkoff sounds.
- Recall the intrinsic factors that influence blood pressure.
- Understand the complications of, and treatment options for, hypertension.
- Describe the factors which influence the tone of vascular smooth muscle.
- Describe the processes involved in solute and fluid transport in capillaries.
- Understand what affects venous and lymphatic flow.
- Understand the factors that regulate blood flow in the vascular beds of specific organs.

HAEMODYNAMICS IN BLOOD VESSELS

Blood flow and velocity

In normal arteries and veins, the pattern of blood flow is described as laminar flow (Fig. 5.1), in which blood flows in a number of parallel planes, with those in the centre flowing faster than those towards the wall of the vessel. This occurs because there is a shear force between layers of blood and the outermost layer of blood and the static wall that causes resistance and slows blood flowing at the periphery of the vessel. Turbulent flow occurs in the ventricles and 'single-file' flow occurs in capillaries where the diameter of the vessel is the same (or often less than) the diameter of red and white blood cells. Although this is a simplistic view, it is sufficient for most basic purposes.

HINTS AND TIPS

Disruption of laminar flow can occur at branching points (e.g. the carotid artery bifurcation) or when there is a narrowing of a vessel. This is important because this disrupted pattern of flow promotes atherosclerosis.

Blood flow is defined as the volume of blood that flows through a given tissue in a given time. Darcy's law (which is equivalent to Ohm's law) states:

$$\text{Flow} = \text{Perfusion pressure/resistance}$$

In a single vascular bed, the blood flow is determined by the arterial pressure minus venous pressure (the perfusion pressure), divided by the resistance to flow in that vascular bed. When considering the circulation as a whole, total blood flow is equal to the cardiac output, and:

$$\text{Cardiac output} = (\text{Mean arterial blood pressure} - \text{central venous pressure})/ \text{systemic vascular resistance}$$

The velocity of blood flow is inversely related to the total cross-sectional area (Fig. 5.2). The branching nature of the circulatory system means that the total cross-sectional area of the capillaries is much greater than that of the large arteries or veins. This substantially reduces velocity in the capillaries, allowing diffusion to take place.

Vascular resistance

Poiseuille's law

Poiseuille determined that resistance (R) to the steady laminar flow of a fluid through a tube is proportional to the length of the tube (l), viscosity of the fluid (η),

53

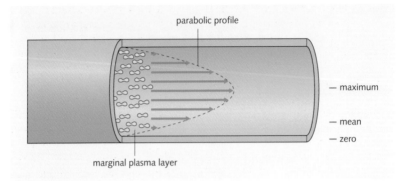

Fig. 5.1 The dynamics of laminar flow. Blood flows as if in sheets (laminae) with blood being faster in the middle than at the sides, where friction slows flow. The dashed line indicates the parabolic profile of the different speeds across the vessel. Cells tend to accumulate in the centre of the flow, leaving a marginal plasma layer with fewer red cells at the periphery.

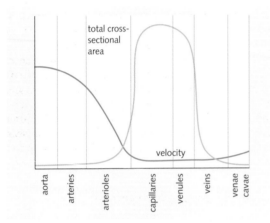

Fig. 5.2 Total cross-sectional area and mean velocity within the different anatomical classifications of vessels. Velocity in the arterial side actually varies during the cardiac cycle – the mean velocity is shown.

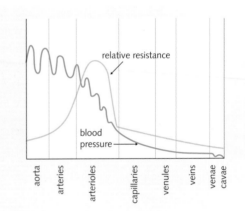

Fig. 5.3 How blood pressure and vascular resistance change across the vascular system. Pressure in the arterial side and in the great veins varies with the cardiac cycle.

and inversely proportional to the fourth power of the radius of the tube (r^4). He stated that:

$$R = 8\eta l/\pi r^4$$

Using Darcy's law we can derive:

$$\text{Flow} = (\text{Pressure difference})/\pi r^4/8\eta l$$

From these equations we can explain the resistance element of Fig. 5.3:

- Total resistance in the vasculature is greatest in the arterioles, through a combination of their length and reduced radius without a significant change in total cross-sectional area.
- Capillary resistance is less than arteriolar resistance because capillaries are shorter (0.5 mm), large numbers of capillaries occur in parallel, and they have single-file flow rather than laminar flow. Remember, however, that due to its smaller radius, a given

length of capillary will have greater resistance than the same length of arteriole.
- Total resistance is dependent upon the arteriolar radius, which is tightly controlled by numerous factors, which are described in detail below.

Blood viscosity

Viscosity, described as 'lack of slipperiness' by Newton, is the measure of the internal friction within a moving fluid. According to Poiseuille's law, resistance is proportional to viscosity and so, the viscosity of the blood plays a role in determining resistance, and therefore flow. The viscosity of blood is influenced by both the plasma and cellular components of blood, but it is the haematocrit (the percentage of red cells in the blood volume) that is the main determinant.

A normal haematocrit value of 47% makes blood viscosity about four times that of water, and is the optimal level for oxygen delivery. An elevated haematocrit increases the carriage of oxygen but increases viscosity, impeding flow and increasing cardiac work. Polycythaemia is the term used to describe an increased haematocrit and can be caused by a physiological adaptation to chronic hypoxia or a myeloproliferative disease increasing red blood cell production by the bone marrow (polycythaemia rubra vera). It may also occur in severe dehydration when circulating volume is reduced without loss of any red blood cells.

Plasma viscosity is determined by the level of plasma proteins (mainly albumins and globulins) and is increased in conditions such as myeloma, in which there is increased production of immunoglobulin. In addition to increasing plasma viscosity, this increase in plasma proteins promotes aggregation of red blood cells, further increasing viscosity. The vessel diameter and the rate of flow also influences red blood cell aggregation and as a result, the viscosity of blood is different at different points in the vascular system.

ARTERIES

The pulse waveform

The waveform of arterial pressure during the cardiac cycle is shown in Fig 5.4:

- During the early part of ventricular ejection, the rate of blood flowing into the aorta is greater than the rate of blood flowing off into the peripheral circulation. This increases the volume of blood in the aorta and thus the pressure. The peak pressure reached is known as the systolic blood pressure (SBP).
- As ejection declines and during diastole, flow from the aorta into the peripheral vessels is greater than flow into the aorta and the pressure drops. The pressure at the end of diastole (which is the lowest in the cycle) is termed diastolic blood pressure (DBP).
- Closure of the aortic valve causes a transient rise in aortic pressure, referred to as the 'dicrotic notch'.

During systole, when aortic pressure increases, the walls of these elastic arteries are stretched and store some of the energy generated by ventricular contraction. They then recoil during diastole to maintain pressure and convert the intermittent flow from the left ventricle into the aorta into more continuous flow into the peripheral vasculature, maintaining perfusion pressure. This stretching and subsequent recoil of the wall of large elastic arteries is known as the Windkessel effect.

Factors that alter the rate of ventricular ejection or outflow from the aorta to the peripheral circulation will alter the shape of the pulse waveform. Aortic stenosis, for example, decreases the rate of ejection and causes what is described as a 'slow rising' pulse while aortic regurgitation, in which blood flows back into the heart through the aortic valve, causes a 'collapsing' pulse. These are shown in Fig. 5.5.

Arterial blood pressure

Arterial blood pressure is determined in the elastic arteries such as the aorta and its major branches, and in the presence of steady venous pressures determines the perfusion pressure for the body's tissues. Arterial blood pressure is expressed as the SBP/DBP.

Measurement of arterial blood pressure

Non-invasive measurement of arterial blood pressure is performed using a sphygmomanometer. In clinical practice it is usually measured using an automatic sphygmomanometer (a machine) but it is important to be able to measure it conventionally with a manual

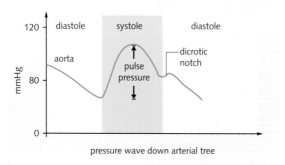

Fig. 5.4 Pulse waveform. The dicrotic notch is caused by closure of the aortic valve.

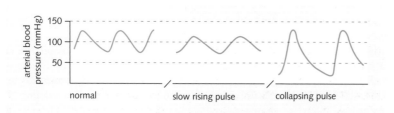

Fig. 5.5 Normal, slow-rising and collapsing pulse waveforms.

sphygmomanometer and a stethoscope. It is also important to appreciate the theory underlying this technique. The sphygmomanometer is used as follows:

1. A suitably sized cuff is wrapped around the upper arm of the patient, who should be sitting or lying with the sphygmomanometer at the level of their heart.
2. The radial or brachial pulse is palpated, and the cuff inflated until the pulse is no longer palpable. This is an estimation of the systolic blood pressure.
3. The brachial artery is auscultated at the medial side of the antecubital fossa with a stethoscope. No sound should be heard.
4. The cuff pressure is gradually lowered (1–2 mmHg/second) until a dull tapping sound is heard. The measurement taken at this time is the systolic pressure.
5. Further lowering of the cuff pressure results in louder sounds until the sounds suddenly become quieter, and then disappear. The measurement taken at this time is the diastolic pressure.

There are a number of audible stages when manually measuring blood pressure, known as the Korotkoff sounds:

I. Sharp thud (taken to be systolic blood pressure).
II. Loud blowing sound.
III. Soft thud.
IV. Soft blowing sound (occasionally used as diastolic blood pressure, e.g. in pregnancy).
V. Onset of silence (taken to be diastolic blood pressure).

Normal blood pressure

Normal blood pressure for a healthy adult male at rest is 120/80 mmHg. However, this value can vary with many factors, all of which must be taken into account when assessing a patient's blood pressure:

- Ageing causes an increase in systolic blood pressure because of decreased arterial compliance secondary to arteriosclerosis. As a rough rule, systolic pressure should be equal to 100 mmHg plus age in years.
- During sleep, blood pressure falls because of the body's decreased metabolic demands.
- Anger, sexual excitement and stress increase blood pressure, all as a result of sympathetically mediated responses.

Other factors that may cause changes in blood pressure include:

- Respiration: in the young, mean arterial pressure falls by a small amount during inspiration because of a transient fall in stroke volume.
- Pregnancy: blood pressure falls gradually in the first trimester, reaching a minimum in the second trimester, and then rises to normal in the third trimester.

Mean arterial blood pressure (mABP)

The mean arterial blood pressure is not simply the average of the systolic and diastolic pressures. It can be estimated using the equation:

$$mABP = DBP + 1/3 \ (SBP - DBP)$$

By rearranging Darcy's law we can deduce:

Mean arterial blood pressure = cardiac output/total peripheral resistance

Cardiac output determines the rate of inflow of blood into the aorta and thus determines the rate at which aortic pressure rises. Total peripheral resistance (TPR) determines the rate of outflow from the aorta and thus the rate at which the pressure drops during diastole. As a rule of thumb, SBP is determined by stroke volume and DBP is determined by TPR. DBP is also affected by heart rate in that as heart rate increases, the duration of diastole shortens and the period in which pressure falls before the onset of systole shortens.

Pulse pressure

The difference between the SBP and the DBP is referred to as the pulse pressure. For a normal BP of 120/80 mmHg, the pulse pressure is 40 mmHg. Pulse pressure can be altered under different circumstances, for example:

- Ageing: as we age, the wall of the aorta becomes less elastic. As a result, there is a greater increase in pressure during ventricular ejection because the walls are less distensible, and thus SBP is higher. DBP, on the other hand, is reduced because the lack of elastic recoil means that pressure drops at a greater rate during diastole. This increases the pulse pressure.
- Haemorrhage: after significant haemorrhage, when blood volume is reduced, stroke volume is usually reduced due to decrease in preload, decreasing SBP. In order to maintain mABP and thus perfusion pressure, TPR is increased, raising DBP and decreasing the pulse pressure. (This example will be discussed further in Ch. 6).
- Aortic valve disease: look at Fig. 5.5. The pulse pressure is decreased in aortic stenosis and increased in aortic regurgitation.

ARTERIOLES

Arterioles are the site of greatest resistance to blood flow in the circulatory system. The abundant smooth muscle in the wall of these vessels allows lumen diameter to be tightly controlled. Contraction of vascular smooth muscle decreases the diameter of the vessel lumen and relaxation increases it. According to Poiseuille's equations, resistance to flow is proportional to the fourth power of the radius. This means that a very small change in lumen radius will have a significant impact of resistance and thus flow.

Control over arteriolar diameter is achieved by a number of tightly regulated mechanisms, which will be discussed in detail below, and has three important functions:

- Coordinated constriction or dilatation of a large proportion of arterioles will alter the total peripheral resistance and thus arterial blood pressure.
- Constriction or dilatation of arterioles in single organs allows the distribution of the cardiac output to different organs to be regulated. Dilatation of the arterioles in a particular organ will decrease resistance and increase flow to that organ.
- Constriction or dilatation of arterioles influences the hydrostatic forces in the capillaries and as a result has an effect on fluid filtration (explained below). Constriction of arterioles increases resistance and causes a greater pressure drop, reducing the pressure in the distal vessels, including the capillaries.

Control of vascular smooth muscle (VSM) tone

Tight control over the arteriolar vascular smooth muscle tone is achieved via numerous mechanisms. Many of the same factors also have an effect on the vascular smooth muscle of the venous capacitance vessels. These mechanisms can be broadly divided into local influences and systemic influences. The mechanisms of VSM contraction and relaxation have been discussed in Chapter 2 but in short, it is important to remember that vasoconstriction is an active process brought about by the contraction of vascular smooth muscle, which as for cardiac muscle requires an increase in cytosolic $[Ca^{2+}]$. Vasodilatation occurs when VSM relaxes and the pressure of blood within the vessel causes it to distend.

Local influences

Myogenic tone

This describes the constrictor response of vascular smooth muscle to stretching of the vessel wall as a result of increased internal pressure. It plays an important role in autoregulation and also contributes to basal tone. The higher the internal hydrostatic pressure, the greater the degree of myogenic constriction.

Endothelium-derived substances

Endothelial cells play an important role in the local regulation of blood flow. Although they do not have a contractile function, they release a number of dilator and constrictor substances, which act on the adjacent smooth muscle cells and influence arteriolar tone.

> The importance of the balance between dilator and constrictor influences on resting VSM can be demonstrated by the administration of a nitric oxide (NO) synthase inhibitor. This causes a 30% increase in blood pressure by increasing total peripheral resistance. This increase is a result of loss of basal release of NO.

Endothelium-derived dilator factors

Endothelium-derived dilating factors include nitric oxide (NO), prostacyclin (PGI2) and endothelium derived hyperpolarizing factor (EDHF). NO is the most important dilator substance. In the endothelium, NO is produced by endothelial nitric oxide synthase (eNOS). eNOS is activated by an increase in intracellular $[Ca^{2+}]$ which can occur in response to factors such as bradykinin, acetylcholine and substance P. It is also activated by the shear forces that are exerted on the endothelial cells by the blood flowing through the vessel. Following its production by eNOS, NO diffuses to the adjacent vascular smooth muscle cells and activates the enzyme guanylyl cyclase increasing levels of cGMP and bringing about dilatation (see Fig. 2.56). In addition to its vasodilator properties, NO has other effects including inhibition of platelet function and inhibition of leukocyte adhesion to the endothelium. Endothelial derived dilator substances, particularly NO, provide a tonic vasodilator effect that counteracts the tonic myogenic vasoconstriction and it is the balance of these that determines the resting tone of the vessel.

Endothelium-derived constrictor factors

Endothelium-derived constricting factors include endothelin 1, thromboxane A_2 and prostaglandin H_2. Endothelin 1 is the most important constrictor released by the endothelium. It is released in response to vasoconstrictor substances including adrenaline/epinephrine, vasopressin and angiotensin II. It then diffuses to the adjacent smooth muscle cells and causes constriction via G-protein coupled mechanisms similar to those activated when noradrenaline/norepinephrine binds to α adrenoceptors (see Fig. 2.54).

Metabolic factors

Locally produced products of metabolism diffuse into the tunica media of the arterioles and cause relaxation of VSM and thus vasodilatation. The amount of these factors released correlates with the local metabolic rate and as a result this process couples blood flow with the metabolic requirements of the tissue and is particularly important in the myocardium and skeletal muscle. The substances responsible for this so called functional or metabolic hyperaemia (increase in blood flow) are not fully established and are different in each organ but candidates include H^+ ions, K^+ ions, hypoxia, adenosine, phosphate ions and prostaglandins.

Another process underpinned by these locally released metabolic factors is that of reactive hyperaemia. This occurs when blood flow is restored to a tissue after a period of interrupted flow, and the amount of blood flowing into the tissue is greater than that under resting conditions, even though there has been no change in the metabolic rate of that tissue. This response is in place to aid removal of metabolic by-products that have accumulated during the period of no flow and to restore oxygen supply as quickly as possible. The effect is temporary and decays exponentially as the metabolic factors are transported away in the blood, reducing their concentration and vasodilator effect.

In both of these processes, metabolites only act on the vascular smooth muscle of the arterioles within that tissue. Although those arterioles are then dilated, in order for blood flow to that tissue to increase, there must also be vasodilatation of the arteries and arterioles upstream that do not necessarily lie within the tissue they supply. This is brought about by a process called flow-mediated vasodilatation in which the shear force (friction of blood against the vessel wall) on the endothelial cells stimulates them to release factors that cause relaxation of adjacent smooth muscle cells.

Other local factors

A number of other substances that are produced, secreted and act locally have an effect on vascular smooth muscle tone. They include:

- Histamine: this is an inflammatory mediator that causes arteriolar vasodilatation (H_1 receptor-mediated). In veins, it causes vasoconstriction and increased permeability (H_2 receptor-mediated).
- Bradykinin: this inflammatory mediator causes endothelium-dependent vasodilatation and increases vascular permeability.
- Thromboxane A_2: this is a platelet activator that causes vasoconstriction; it is involved in haemostasis.
- Leukotrienes: these are inflammatory mediators synthesized from arachidonic acid by the enzyme lipoxygenase. They are produced by leukocytes, and cause vasoconstriction and increased vascular permeability.
- Platelet activating factor (PAF): this is an inflammatory mediator that causes vasodilatation and increased vascular permeability.

The net effect of these inflammatory mediators is vasodilatation and increased vascular permeability.

These changes bring about redness, warmth and swelling (due to oedema), three of the characteristic features of inflammation.

Systemic influences

The local influences described above serve only the needs of the local tissues without taking into account the requirements of the whole body, including maintenance of blood pressure. Consider a situation in which all the tissues in the body had increased requirements and thus local factors brought about vasodilatation in all the tissues simultaneously. This would cause a massive decrease in total peripheral resistance, decreasing blood pressure. In order to maintain blood pressure, the central nervous system exerts effects on vascular tone that are superimposed on those local factors. There are also hormonal factors that act systemically to influence vascular tone.

Autonomic nervous influences

Sympathetic vasoconstrictor nerves

Sympathetic vasoconstrictor nerves innervate the vascular smooth muscle of the arterioles and of the venous vessels. In arterioles, a basal level of activity of these nerves is partly responsible for vessel tone at rest. The neurotransmitter involved is noradrenaline/norepinephrine, which acts on α_1 receptors on vascular smooth muscle causing contraction. This contraction is brought about by a G-protein coupled response that increases cytosolic $[Ca^{2+}]$ in the VSM cells in response to binding of noradrenaline/norepinephrine. A decrease in sympathetic nerve activity has the opposite effect, and causes relaxation of VSM and vasodilatation.

> Under normal circumstances in most vascular beds, it is decreased activity of sympathetic nerves acting on α_1 adrenoceptors that brings about vasodilatation, not increased activity on β_2 receptors.

The amount of neurotransmitter released is primarily dependent on the degree of sympathetic activity but it is also modulated by other factors. These include locally produced metabolites including adenosine and K^+ that decrease the amount of noradrenaline/norepinephrine released. Angiotensin II has the opposite effect, increasing noradrenaline/norepinephrine release and augmenting vasoconstriction.

HINTS AND TIPS

It is important to remember sympathetic activity to different parts of the body can be adjusted independently. It is not an all or nothing system.

Sympathetic vasodilator nerves

In some species (though not humans), some tissues, including skeletal muscle, are also innervated by sympathetic vasodilator nerves. In humans, this sympathetic dilator innervation is only present in the sweat glands. In skeletal muscle, vascular bed stimulation by these nerves (which use acetylcholine as the neurotransmitter and act on muscarinic receptors) causes vasodilatation. Stimulation only occurs as part of an 'alerting response', and it is initiated in the forebrain without any brainstem influence. The vasodilator effect is only temporary, and it plays no role in blood pressure regulation. Stimulation of these nerves in sweat glands, probably also involving vasoactive intestinal peptide (VIP) as a neurotransmitter, brings about sweating and cutaneous vasodilatation.

Parasympathetic vasodilator nerves

Parasympathetic vasodilator nerves innervate the blood vessels of the:

- Genitalia.
- Skin.
- Salivary glands.
- Pancreas.
- Gastrointestinal mucosa.

The neurotransmitters involved include acetylcholine, VIP and the potent vasodilator nitric oxide. The effect of these nerves on the total peripheral resistance is small because of their limited innervation. These nerves are crucial for initiating an erection. Upon stimulation they produce a vasodilatation in the arterioles supplying the corpus cavernosum of the penis. This increases blood flow into the penis.

Hormonal influences

Although the vasculature is influenced by circulating hormones, short-term control is primarily achieved by the autonomic nervous system under basal conditions. Many of these hormones (except catecholamines) have an important role in regulation of fluid excretion in the kidneys as well as effects on vascular tone.

Catecholamines

The catecholamines (adrenaline/epinephrine and noradrenaline/norepinephrine) are secreted from the adrenal medulla.

More than three times as much adrenaline/epinephrine is secreted as noradrenaline/norepinephrine; however, plasma levels of noradrenaline/norepinephrine are higher than adrenaline/epinephrine due to spillover from sympathetic nerve terminals. Secretion of both catecholamines is increased in response to exercise, hypotension and stressful 'fight or flight' situations.

Both adrenaline/epinephrine and noradrenaline/norepinephrine bind β_1 receptors in the myocardium, increasing heart rate and contractility, and bind α_1 adrenoceptors on vascular smooth muscle causing vasoconstriction, but their affinities for these receptors differ. Adrenaline/epinephrine, but not noradrenaline/norepinephrine, has a high affinity for β_2 receptors, which are present in skeletal muscle and the myocardium. Binding of adrenaline/epinephrine to these receptors brings about vasodilatation. Circulating catecholamines do not have as great an effect as noradrenaline/norepinephrine released from sympathetic nerve terminals because the neurally released noradrenaline/norepinephrine is specifically targeted at the appropriate receptors.

> **HINTS AND TIPS**
>
> Remember adrenaline/epinephrine does not cause vasodilatation in all tissues, only those that express β_2 receptors. Even in these tissues, it still binds α receptors, but the dilator effect of β receptor activation predominates.

Antidiuretic hormone (ADH)

ADH (also called vasopressin) is a peptide produced in the hypothalamus and released from the posterior pituitary directly into the bloodstream. A rise in plasma osmolality is the main stimulus for secretion. Falling blood pressure and angiotensin II are also stimuli for ADH release, but to a lesser degree. ADH promotes water retention in the renal tubules and high levels of ADH also cause vasoconstriction in most tissues. The cerebral and coronary vessels, in contrast, demonstrate a nitric oxide-mediated dilatation in response to ADH.

Angiotensin II

Renin is an enzyme produced by the juxtaglomerular cells of the kidney. It converts circulating angiotensinogen to angiotensin I (Fig. 5.6). Renin production is increased by:

- A fall in afferent arteriolar hydrostatic pressure which supplies the renal glomeruli.
- Increased sympathetic activity to the renal arterioles.
- Binding of adrenaline/epinephrine to β_1 receptors in the kidney.
- Decreased Na^+ in the macula densa of the adjacent distal tubule.

Angiotensin-converting enzyme (ACE) converts angiotensin I to the peptide angiotensin II (Fig. 5.6), predominantly on the endothelium of the pulmonary vascular bed. Angiotensin II is the active component

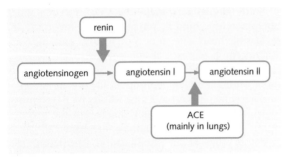

Fig. 5.6 Formation of angiotensin II. Angiotensinogen is secreted by the liver, acted on by renin (secreted by the kidney) and finally converted to the active angiotensin II by angiotensin-converting enzyme (ACE).

of this so-called renin–angiotensin system (RAS) and has the following actions:

- Increases aldosterone secretion from the adrenal cortex, leading to salt and water reabsorption in the distal tubules of the kidneys.
- Causes vasoconstriction by acting directly on vascular smooth muscle, augmenting release of noradrenaline/norepinephrine from sympathetic nerve terminals, and increasing sympathetic outflow from the brainstem.
- Stimulates release of ADH from the posterior pituitary.

Natriuretic peptides

In response to high cardiac filling pressures, specialized myocytes in the atria secrete atrial natriuretic peptide (ANP) as they are stretched. In a similar manner, ventricular myocytes secrete brain natriuretic peptide (BNP) in response to stretch. These natriuretic peptides increase the excretion of salt and water in renal tubules and have a mild vasodilator effect.

Autoregulation

Autoregulation is the process whereby tissue perfusion remains relatively constant across a range of perfusion pressures. This helps to keep capillary filtration pressure at a stable value. Autoregulation is central to regulation of blood flow in the cerebral circulation but is not present in most vascular beds.

Flow is determined by perfusion pressure and resistance. Therefore, to keep flow constant, any change in perfusion pressure must be matched by a change in resistance. An increase in perfusion pressure causes arteriolar vasoconstriction, thereby increasing resistance. Likewise, a decrease in perfusion pressure causes arteriolar vasodilatation and decreases resistance. It takes roughly 30–60 seconds for the effect to take place so

there is an initial increase in flow with a pressure increase before a steady state is reached.

Autoregulation only occurs over a limited pressure range, and if perfusion pressure drops below the autoregulatory range or increases beyond it, blood flow cannot be maintained at its set level. It is an intrinsic feature of the vessels, and it is independent of nervous control. However, it does not mean that tissue perfusion is constant all the time in vivo. Autoregulation can be reset to work at a new level by, for example, an increased sympathetic drive. The mechanisms for autoregulation include:

- Myogenic response: described above.
- Vasodilator washout: this idea is based on the effect of blood flow on the levels of locally produced metabolites. When blood flow increases, there is greater removal of vasodilator metabolites allowing the arterioles to constrict and restoring flow to its set level.

HYPERTENSION

Current British Hypertension Society guidelines define hypertension as a sustained resting blood pressure above 140 mmHg systolic and/or 90 mmHg diastolic. These criteria, however, are somewhat arbitrary as blood pressure rises with age and levels are variable within populations. Cardiovascular disease risk increases with increasing blood pressure, even within the normal range.

Classification and causes

Hypertension is classified according to its underlying cause. Primary (essential) hypertension accounts for 95% of hypertensive patients; the precise aetiology is unknown, but it is probably multifactorial. Remember that to have an increase in blood pressure there must be an increase in cardiac output, total peripheral resistance or both. Predisposing factors include:

- Age (blood pressure rises with age).
- Obesity.
- Excessive alcohol intake.
- High salt intake.
- Genetic susceptibility.

Secondary hypertension accounts for the remaining 5% of cases. Here, the hypertension arises as a result of another disease process. Causes of secondary hypertension include:

- Renal: parenchymal damage can cause an increase in BP. Atherosclerosis in the renal arteries causing renal artery stenosis also causes hypertension by decreasing renal perfusion stimulating the renin–angiotensin system.

- Endocrine.
  - Conn's syndrome (primary hyperaldosteronism): causes salt and water retention, increasing blood volume, preload and therefore cardiac output.
  - Phaeochromocytoma: catecholamine–releasing tumour of the adrenal medulla.
- Coarctation of the aorta: a narrowing of the aorta, usually just distal to the left subclavian vein increases resistance to flow through the aorta, thus increasing total peripheral resistance and blood pressure.
- Pregnancy: hypertension occurs during 10% of first pregnancies.
- Drugs: the oral contraceptive pill causes hypertension in approximately 5% of women.

Malignant hypertension

In this condition, blood pressure rises rapidly to very high levels with the diastolic pressure exceeding 130–140 mmHg. It is more common in secondary hypertension, especially phaeochromocytoma, and it causes rapid development of end-organ damage.

> **HINTS AND TIPS**
>
> The distinction between primary and secondary hypertension is of great clinical significance, since only in the latter case is treatment of the underlying cause possible. The younger the patients and the less risk factors that are present, the more effort that should be made to find an underlying cause.

Complications of hypertension

- Atherosclerosis: hypertension increases the risk of developing clinically significant atherosclerotic plaques. This increases the risk of stroke, peripheral vascular disease and myocardial infarction.
- Renal damage: gradual development of renal dysfunction occurs in hypertension, especially if it is poorly controlled. The pattern of renal disease caused by hypertension is often referred to as hypertensive nephrosclerosis.
- Cardiac: the increased afterload caused by the raised blood pressure increases left ventricular work and causes left ventricular hypertrophy. This can lead to heart failure.
- Arrhythmia: the risk of atrial fibrillation is increased in hypertensive individuals.
- Retinal damage: retinal haemorrhages and papilloedema (in advanced stages) cause visual disturbances.

Note that hypertension itself is usually asymptomatic, and in essential hypertension no obvious cause can be found. This can affect compliance with therapy, especially if drugs have unwanted side-effects.

Effects of hypertension of the vessels

Hypertension not only accelerates atherosclerosis, but it also results in characteristic changes to arterioles and small arteries – known as arteriolosclerosis. All these changes are associated with narrowing of the vessel lumen. Changes in benign hypertension include:

- In arteries: muscular hypertrophy of the media, re-duplication of the external lamina and intimal thickening.
- In arterioles: hyaline arteriosclerosis (protein deposits in wall).
- In vessels of the brain: microaneurysms (Charcot–Bouchard aneurysms) can occur.

Antihypertensive drugs

Angiotensin-converting enzyme inhibitors

Angiotensin-converting enzyme (ACE) inhibitors (e.g. captopril, enalapril, perindopril) inhibit the conversion of angiotensin I to angiotensin II by ACE (Fig. 5.7). They also inhibit bradykinin (a vasodilator) breakdown by ACE. Side-effects include first dose hypotension, a skin rash and a dry cough (in approximately 10%). They should not be used to treat patients with severe renal artery stenosis because inhibition of angiotensin II production will prevent the efferent arteriolar constriction that maintains glomerular filtration in the presence of renal artery stenosis.

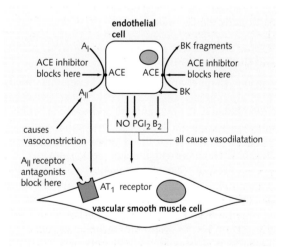

Fig. 5.7 Action of angiotensin-converting enzyme (ACE) inhibitors and angiotensin II (A_{II}) receptor antagonists (A_I, angiotensin I; A_{II}, angiotensin II; AT_1, angiotensin II receptor type 1; B_2, activated bradykinin-activated by endothelial cell; BK, bradykinin; NO, nitric oxide; PGI_2, prostacyclin).

Angiotensin II receptor antagonists

Angiotensin II receptor antagonists (e.g. losartan) inhibit angiotensin II from binding to its receptor. They are useful when ACE inhibitors have produced an intolerable cough (caused by elevated bradykinin).

Diuretics

Usually a thiazide-type diuretic is used (e.g. bendroflumethiazide). These drugs inhibit sodium reabsorption in the distal renal tubule, which causes increased salt and water excretion, decreasing blood volume and thus decreasing blood pressure. Although loop diuretics (e.g. furosemide) produce a more marked diuresis, they are not used in hypertension. Thiazide diuretics also have a direct vasodilator effect, further reducing blood pressure. The important side-effect to be aware of is hypokalaemia, which increases the risk of arrhythmia.

Alpha-blockers

Alpha-blockers (e.g. prazosin and doxazosin) are antagonists of α adrenoceptors. There is postsynaptic blockade of α_1 adrenoceptors, which prevents sympathetically mediated VSM contraction and leads to vasodilatation. They cause a decrease in total peripheral resistance and thus a decrease in blood pressure. Doxazosin is often used for labile (catecholamine-mediated) hypertension. Blockade of α receptors also prevents sympathetically mediated release of renin in the kidneys.

Side-effects of alpha-blockers include postural hypotension caused by loss of sympathetic vasoconstriction, particularly marked following the first dose.

Calcium channel blockers

Calcium channel antagonists (e.g. verapamil, nifedipine, amlodipine, diltiazem) block voltage-gated calcium channels in myocardium and vascular smooth muscle. This causes a decrease in myocardial contractility, electrical conductance and vascular tone. Calcium antagonists interfere with the action of various vasoconstrictor agonists (e.g. noradrenaline/norepinephrine, angiotensin II, thrombin). Verapamil predominantly acts on the heart and decreases heart rate by causing an inhibition of conduction through the AV node. It also acts on the myocardium exerting a negative inotropic effect. It should be used only very cautiously with beta-blockers as this may lead to heart block. Nifedipine and amlodipine (dihydropiridines) act peripherally on arterioles, relaxing arteriolar vascular smooth muscle and causing vasodilatation. These dihydropiridine calcium channel blockers do not slow the heart rate. Diltiazem acts both on the heart and on the arterioles.

> The targets and effects of the different calcium channel blockers:
> - Verapamil: acts on myocardial and AV nodal cells decreasing heart rate and decreasing contractility.
> - Diltiazem: acts on the heart and arterioles decreasing heart rate and causing vasodilatation.
> - Amlodipine and nifedipine: act on arterioles causing vasodilatation.

Beta-blockers

Beta-blockers are antagonists of β adrenoceptors. They block sympathetic activity in the heart (β_1), peripheral vasculature (β_2) and other tissues including the bronchi (β_2). In the heart, this results in a decrease in heart rate and myocardial contractility, which reduces cardiac output and blood pressure.

The effect of beta-blockers on the peripheral vasculature leads to a loss of β-mediated vasodilatation causing an unopposed α vasoconstriction. This may initially cause an increase in vascular resistance, elevating blood pressure, but, in long-term use, the vascular resistance returns to pretreatment levels. Some beta-blockers can preferentially act on β_1 adrenoceptors, being more cardioselective; however, even these drugs have some blocking effect on the β_2 adrenoceptor. Types of beta-blockers include:

- Propranolol, atenolol (act on β_1, β_2).
- Metoprolol, bisoprolol (selective β_1 blockers).

The main side-effects of beta-blockers are bronchoconstriction and bradycardia. They should therefore not be used in people with asthma or chronic obstructive pulmonary disease as they may exacerbate symptoms.

Choice of drugs

The choice of antihypertensive agents in newly diagnosed patients should be guided by the British Hypertension Society algorithm, shown in Fig. 5.8.

CAPILLARIES

In most tissues, groups of capillaries (often referred to as a capillary unit) are supplied by a single terminal arteriole, and the tone of the vascular smooth muscle in that arteriole determines the perfusion of that capillary unit. In certain vascular beds, such as the mesenteric circulation, capillaries branch from vessels that run directly

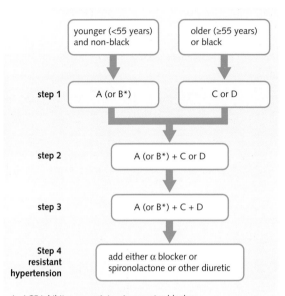

A: ACE inhibitor or angiotensin receptor blocker
B: β blocker
C: calcium channel blocker
D: diuretic (thiazide and thiazide-like)

* combination therapy involving B and D may induce more new onset diabetes compared with other combination therapies

Fig. 5.8 British Hypertension Society guidelines for management of hypertension.

from small arterioles to venules. Blood flow through these capillaries is regulated by small rings of smooth muscle called 'pre-capillary sphincters' (Fig. 5.9). The vascular smooth muscle in these microvessels has relatively sparse innervation and the tone is predominantly controlled by

local factors such as those described above. Under normal conditions, tone in these terminal arterioles and pre-capillary sphincters fluctuates between constriction and dilatation, a process termed vasomotion. This means that blood flow through capillaries is intermittent as the perfusion pressure for individual capillary units is altered. Changes in terminal arteriolar diameter and capillary perfusion pressure also have an impact on fluid filtration (explained below).

Capillary diameter is often smaller than red blood cell diameter (3–6 μm compared with 8–10 μm), but because the red blood cells can deform they are still able to pass through the microvasculature. Under certain pathological conditions such as sickle cell anaemia, red blood cells become more rigid as the concentration of oxygen decreases in the blood (as occurs during capillary transit) and can cause obstruction of the microvasculature, precipitating a vaso-occlusive crisis.

Solute exchange

Exchange of solutes in the microvasculature generally occurs by diffusion down concentration gradients. The processes involved are depicted in Fig. 5.10 and include:

1. Diffusion through the endothelial cells: lipid-soluble substances such as oxygen and carbon dioxide diffuse through the endothelial cell lipid membranes and into the extracellular space. The rate of diffusion is governed by Fick's law, which states that diffusion equals the diffusion constant of the barrier (i.e. the capillary wall), multiplied by the surface area available for diffusion and the concentration gradient of the substance.

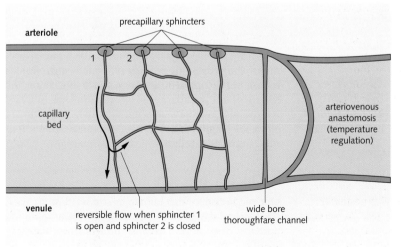

Fig. 5.9 Capillary circulation. Flow may be reversible in some vessels (vasomotion) depending on the closure of the precapillary sphincters.

Fig. 5.10 The various mechanisms of capillary transport.

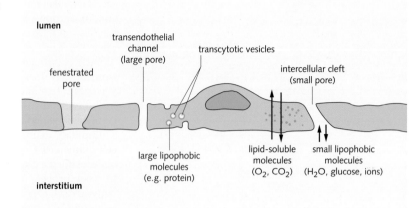

2. Diffusion through pores and fenestrations in the capillary wall: water and water-soluble substances (e.g. glucose, amino acids, ions) diffuse through small 'pores' that constitute the intercellular clefts between endothelial cells. This process is also called bulk flow. The degree of bulk flow varies in different organs depending on the structure of the capillaries (see Ch. 2). Vascular beds with continuous capillaries limit bulk flow while some vascular beds such as the exocrine glands, liver and spleen have large gaps in the capillary wall (due to their fenestrated or discontinuous structure), have a relatively high permeability and allow greater bulk flow. There are also a few large pores for larger molecules, especially in the liver and spleen where the endothelial cells are discontinuous. In the brain, the endothelial cell junctions have a complex arrangement of fibres that make them impermeable to lipophobic molecules. This comprises the blood–brain barrier, which tightly controls transport of molecules in and out of the brain.

3. Vesicular transport.
   Some molecules (e.g. plasma proteins) are transported across the endothelial cell by transcytotic vesicles. Unlike the processes already described that are all passive, this is an active transport process requiring energy.

HINTS AND TIPS

Diffusion of oxygen can be enhanced by increased blood concentration, increased blood flow, increased surface area, or decreased tissue oxygen concentration. For carbon dioxide, the diffusion constant is much higher and diffusion is limited by blood flow alone.

Fluid exchange

When considering fluid exchange in the microcirculation, consider two compartments. The intravascular (capillary) compartment and the interstitial (tissue) compartment (the two components of the extracellular fluid). Fluid can freely pass between the intravascular compartment of the capillaries and post-capillary venules and the interstitial space around them by bulk flow. This movement of fluid, termed fluid filtration, is governed by two opposing forces according to Starling's hypothesis of tissue fluid formation.

1. Hydrostatic pressure

Hydrostatic pressure is the pressure exerted on the wall of a vessel by the fluid within. The net hydrostatic pressure is the difference between the hydrostatic in the intravascular space (capillary hydrostatic pressure, CHP) and the hydrostatic pressure in the interstitial fluid (tissue hydrostatic pressure, THP). Capillary hydrostatic pressure is typically 37 mmHg at the arterial end of the capillary and 17 mmHg at the venous end, falling steadily along the length of the vessel. The pressure at the arterial end will vary with the vasomotion that results from changes in vascular tone in the terminal arterioles. The hydrostatic pressure of the interstitial fluid is low, around 2 mmHg and remains stable along the length of the capillary. As a result the net outward hydrostatic pressure falls from 35 mmHg to 15 mmHg along the length of the capillary and causes filtration of fluid from the capillaries into the interstitium.

2. Oncotic pressure

Oncotic pressure (also known as colloid osmotic pressure) is determined by the concentration of large plasma proteins that cannot usually diffuse across capillary walls. The significantly larger concentrations of these within the plasma results in a capillary oncotic pressure of around 25 mmHg and a tissue (interstitial) oncotic pressure of 1 mmHg. These forces cause a net movement of fluid (reabsorption) from the interstitium into the vascular space because water always moves by osmosis from areas of low solute concentration to areas of high solute concentration. Effectively, the net oncotic pressure pulls fluid from the interstitial compartment into the capillaries. This remains relatively constant along the length of the vessel. If the permeability of the capillary wall to large molecules is increased, however, plasma proteins will diffuse into the interstitium and there will be an increase in tissue oncotic pressure, decreasing the net oncotic pressure. Such an increase in capillary permeability occurs in response to release of local inflammatory mediators such as histamine, bradykinin and leukotrienes.

Net filtration

The net movement of fluid in or out of the capillary at any one point depends on the balance of the net hydrostatic pressure and net oncotic pressure. At the arterial end of the capillary a net filtration of fluid (out of the capillary) occurs, whereas at the venous end a net reabsorption (into the capillary) takes place (Fig. 5.11). Under basal conditions in the body as a whole, approximately 20 L of fluid is filtered out of the capillaries and 16 L reabsorbed into the capillaries every 24 h. This net loss from the vascular space is returned via the lymphatic system. The balance of these forces and thus the net amount of fluid filtration is influenced by a number of factors, some of which are illustrated in Fig. 5.12.

If a large amount of fluid is filtered into the interstitial space and the lymphatic drainage is not sufficient to remove it, it causes swelling of the tissue known as oedema. This often occurs in the ankles where the capillary hydrostatic pressure is greatest due to the effect of gravity. Fluid filtration in the pulmonary circulation is of great importance. Excessive filtration of fluid into the interstitium, termed pulmonary oedema, restricts gas exchange in the alveoli and can cause respiratory failure. This can occur when pulmonary venous pressures are raised in left ventricular heart failure, or when there is a large local or systemic inflammatory response during which vascular permeability is increased, increasing tissue oncotic pressure.

Distribution of the lymphatic tissues

Fluid, proteins and fat globules not reabsorbed into capillaries are brought back into the vascular system through the lymphatic system (Fig. 5.13). There is a network of lymphatic capillaries, ducts, and lymph nodes that drain excess tissue/interstitial fluid and unite to form the thoracic duct, which drains the collected fluid into the left subclavian vein. There are certain specialized areas of lymphatic tissue associated with the immune response but these are beyond the scope of this book.

Fluid and proteins in the interstitial space are driven into the lymphatic capillaries by the hydrostatic pressure of the interstitial fluid (tissue hydrostatic pressure). Lymph is moved along the lymphatics by smooth muscle contractions in the vessel wall, which increase with volume, and extrinsic propulsion by the skeletal muscle pump and intestinal peristalsis. Backflow is prevented by the presence of valves.

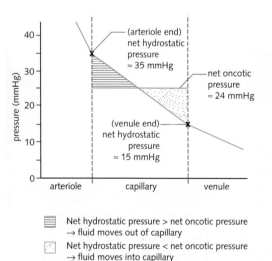

Net hydrostatic pressure > net oncotic pressure
→ fluid moves out of capillary

Net hydrostatic pressure < net oncotic pressure
→ fluid moves into capillary

Fig. 5.11 The hydrostatic and oncotic pressures influencing capillary filtration.

> ### HINTS AND TIPS
>
> The lymphatics are the mopping up system of the body, taking up any excess filtrate and returning it to the main circulatory system. They also carry foreign antigens from the blood to cells of the immune system located in the lymph nodes.

Fig. 5.12 Factors that alter capillary fluid filtration.

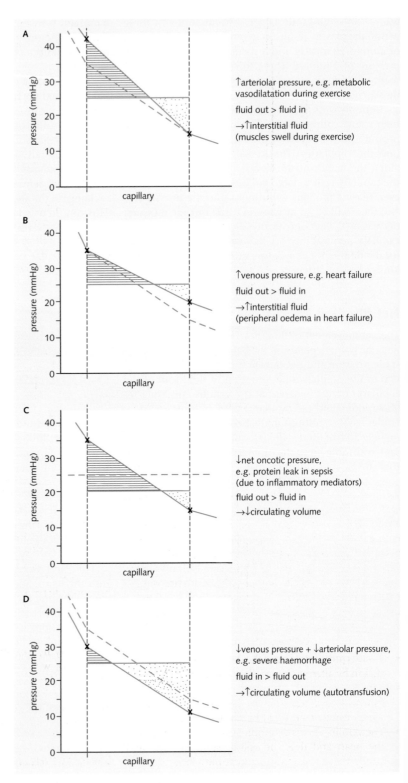

A

↑arteriolar pressure, e.g. metabolic vasodilatation during exercise

fluid out > fluid in

→↑interstitial fluid
(muscles swell during exercise)

B

↑venous pressure, e.g. heart failure

fluid out > fluid in

→↑interstitial fluid
(peripheral oedema in heart failure)

C

↓net oncotic pressure,
e.g. protein leak in sepsis
(due to inflammatory mediators)

fluid out > fluid in

→↓circulating volume

D

↓venous pressure + ↓arteriolar pressure,
e.g. severe haemorrhage

fluid in > fluid out

→↑circulating volume (autotransfusion)

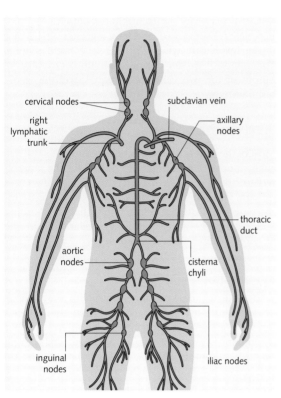

cervical nodes

subclavian vein

right lymphatic trunk

axillary nodes

aortic nodes

thoracic duct

cisterna chyli

inguinal nodes

iliac nodes

Fig. 5.13 Lymphatic drainage of the body. The lymphatics drain into the left and right subclavian veins.

VEINS AND VENULES

Venules and veins are thin-walled, distensible vessels that return blood from the capillaries to the right atrium, but to think of them merely as passive conduits is to greatly underestimate their importance. One important feature of venous vessels is the presence of valves. These valves prevent backflow of blood within the veins and are crucial because without them, venous return would be limited. The effects of valve failure in the lower limbs can be illustrated by the occurrence of varicose veins (described in Ch. 9). Venous vessels have other important functions and influences:

- Venous pressure is one of the determinants of fluid filtration by altering the capillary hydrostatic pressure.
- Due to their high compliance, venous vessels can function as a reservoir for blood, the volume of which can be controlled by numerous factors.
- The venous vessels determine the filling pressures of the heart and thus the end-diastolic volume and stroke volume according to Starling's law.

The pressure in the veins (venous pressure) depends on the volume of blood they contain and the state of the smooth muscle in their walls and is extremely important because it determines the venous return to the

heart and thus right ventricular end-diastolic volume. These factors can be affected by both passive influences and active influences. Always try and think of the forward (central venous pressure and cardiac filling pressures) and backward (capillary hydrostatic pressure) effects of changes in venous volume and pressure. Look back to Fig. 2.49 to review the relationship between volume and pressure in venous vessels.

Passive influences

Blood volume

As explained in Chapter 2, venous vessels are very compliant up to a point, at which pressure increases quickly with further increases in volume. When blood volume increases, there is an increase in venous pressure, which increases both capillary hydrostatic pressure and central venous pressure.

Posture

Venous pressures when supine are:

- 12–20 mmHg in venules.
- 8–10 mmHg in the femoral vein.
- 0–6 mmHg in the central veins and right atrium.

Although these pressures are small, resistance is also small, and the pressure is sufficient to drive blood into the right atrium. Orthostasis (the movement from supine to standing) increases blood pressure in any vessel below heart level and decreases pressure in any vessel above. This is caused by the effect of gravity on the column of blood in the vessel. It is important to remember that the effect of gravity occurs in venous and arterial vessels alike. The increase in pressure in arteries and veins is equal so although the absolute pressures increase, the perfusion pressure remains the same, maintaining tissue perfusion and not impeding the return of blood to the heart. The increase in venous pressure does, however, distend the veins resulting in a degree of venous pooling (approximately 500 mL), which causes a decrease in cardiac output because of an 'apparent' reduction in circulating volume. There is also an increase in capillary hydrostatic pressure (both arterial and venous end), which increases net filtration of fluid out of the vascular compartment, decreasing circulating volume. These changes do not usually cause prolonged haemodynamic changes because compensatory mechanisms are in place (explained in Ch. 6).

Skeletal muscle pump

Rhythmic exercise, especially of the leg muscles, produces a pumping effect increasing movement of venous blood into the central veins, maintaining venous return (Fig. 5.14). By pumping blood out of the active muscle,

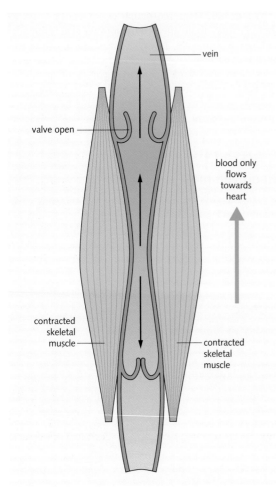

Fig. 5.14 Skeletal muscle pump. Contraction of the surrounding muscle drives the blood towards the heart. It is prevented from returning by the closure of venous valves.

this muscle pump lowers the venous pressure in that muscle, increasing perfusion pressure and increasing blood flow through active muscles. It also decreases capillary hydrostatic pressure at the venous end of capillary units, thereby reducing muscle swelling. Incompetent venous valves will make the skeletal muscle pump ineffective. Static exercise (rather than dynamic), does not act as a pump, but it does increase central venous pressure because it prevents venous pooling by compressing the veins.

Respiratory pump

During inspiration, there is a decrease in intrathoracic pressure and an increase in intra-abdominal pressure as the diaphragm descends. This causes a rise in blood flow into the thorax, increasing right-sided filling pressures and stroke volume. Left ventricular stroke volume,

however, decreases on inspiration because the pulmonary veins are stretched, and have a greater capacitance during inspiration, which reduces left ventricular filling. The opposite occurs during expiration. Overall, the output of the two ventricles is equal over the whole respiratory cycle.

Active influences

Most of the factors described above that control the vascular smooth muscle of the arterioles have the same effect on the VSM of veins. There are some differences though: for example, angiotensin II does not have a direct constrictor effect on veins, unlike that on arterioles, and histamine, which causes vasodilatation in the arterioles, causes constriction of veins.

Sympathetic innervation

Veins (not venules) are innervated with sympathetic noradrenergic nerves. When stimulated these nerves release noradrenaline/norepinephrine at the vascular smooth muscle which causes venoconstriction by acting on α adrenoceptors. This increases venous pressure and reduces venous pooling, increasing venous return.

Circulating catecholamines

Circulating noradrenaline/norepinephrine and adrenaline/epinephrine can cause venoconstriction by acting on α adrenoceptors on venous smooth muscle.

REGULATION OF BLOOD FLOW IN SPECIFIC TISSUES

Fig. 5.15 shows the proportion of blood flow received by the major organs of the body. Although the major vascular beds of the body share many characteristics, they have a number of adaptations that make them better suited to their function.

Coronary circulation

Myocardial oxygen demand is very high, being about 8 mL O_2/min/100 g, and can increase up to five-fold during exercise. Even at rest, the coronary circulation receives 3–5% of the total cardiac output, 10 times the average blood flow per gram of tissue. Oxygen levels in coronary venous blood are very low (due to high oxygen extraction, >70%), so an increase in demand can only be met by increasing arterial flow. During systole, coronary artery branches in the myocardium are compressed by the high transmural pressure gradients across the myocardium, partially impeding blood flow. These

Fig. 5.15 Distribution of cardiac output to the various systems of the body

Organ	Mass (kg)	Blood flow (mL/min)	Blood flow per 100 g (mL/min/100 g)	Proportion of cardiac output (%)
Brain	1.4	750	54.0	13.9 [18.4]
Heart	0.3	250	84.0	4.7 [11.6]
Liver	1.5	1500*	100.0*	27.8 [20.4]*
(Gastrointestinal tract)	(2.5)	(1170)	(46.8)	(21.7 [16.0])
Kidneys	0.3	1260	420	23.3 [7.2]
Skeletal muscle	31.0	840	2.7	15.6 [20.0]
Skin	3.6	460	12.8	8.6 [4.8]
Rest of body	22.4	340	1.5	6.1 [17.6]
Whole body	63.0	5400	8.6	100 [100]

Note that the blood flow to the gastrointestinal tract (shown in round brackets) also flows through the liver via the portal circulation. Values for the liver marked * include the portal and arterial circulation to the liver. Values in square brackets denote the percentage of oxygen consumption by the various systems.

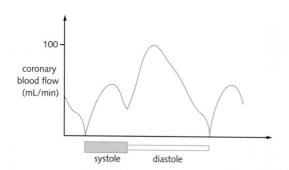

Fig. 5.16 Coronary blood flow during the cardiac cycle. Note that maximal blood flow is during diastole.

pressures are decreased during diastole and flow is restored. This is important to remember because situations where heart rate in increased, decreases the duration of diastole and thus the time for maximal coronary blood flow (Fig. 5.16).

Oxygen transport is aided by the high capillary density (large area and decreased distance for exchange). Blood flow is primarily controlled by local tissue levels of the vasodilator adenosine which is produced from the breakdown of ATP when the local concentration of oxygen is decreased. An increase in the levels of adenosine produces a metabolic hyperaemia, increasing blood flow and oxygen delivery. Sympathetic α_1 noradrenergic vasoconstriction can occur but this is overcome by the local metabolic vasodilator influences.

Coronary arteries are functional end arteries with few cross-connections between them. This means that if they are occluded, there is a limited collateral blood supply and perfusion to that area is almost abolished.

Cerebral circulation

Grey matter has a high oxygen consumption and accounts for approximately 20% of total body oxygen consumption at rest. As grey matter has very little tolerance to hypoxia, consciousness is lost after a few seconds of ischaemia and thus one of the primary functions of the cardiovascular system is to maintain an adequate supply of oxygen to the brain. Autoregulation is crucial and well developed in the cerebral circulation (see page 62), but this eventually fails when pressure falls below 50 mmHg or exceeds 170 mmHg. Cerebral vessels are very sensitive to arterial P_{CO_2}:

- Hypercapnia causes vasodilatation (Fig. 5.17).
- Hypocapnia causes vasoconstriction.

Reduction in arterial P_{CO_2} through hyperventilation can lead to cerebral vasoconstriction, and even transient unconsciousness. This is why people who are hyperventilating are often told to rebreathe air in and out of a paper bag, to prevent development of hypocapnia. Cerebral vessels do not participate in baroreflex vasoconstriction.

Autoregulation sets the total amount of blood flow that enters the cerebral circulation but mechanisms must be in place to ensure that blood is directed to the metabolically active areas of the brain. This process

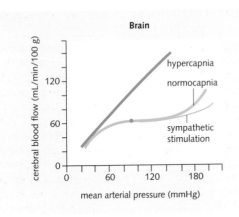

Fig. 5.17 Pressure–flow curves for the cerebral vasculature showing autoregulation at normal arterial P_{CO_2} and the effect of hypercapnia.

is called flow-metabolism coupling and is extremely precise. The precise mechanism underlying this is not known but substances involved include K^+ ions, the neurotransmitter glutamate and products of arachidonic acid metabolism.

In young people, the circle of Willis enables blood supply to be maintained if one carotid artery is occluded. These anastomoses linking the arteries together are less effective in the elderly. The presence of a blood–brain barrier (BBB) tightly controls the neuronal environment allowing lipid-soluble molecules to diffuse freely, but not diffusion of ionic solutes. Transport of water is tightly controlled by the BBB. This is a crucial function, as excessive water within the cerebral interstitium will cause swelling of the brain, and because the brain is enclosed within a rigid container (the skull) this increases intracranial pressure.

Pulmonary circulation

The entire output of the right ventricle enters the pulmonary circulation. A separate bronchial circulation arising from the descending aorta meets the metabolic needs of the bronchi and smaller airways. There is a very high capillary density and a very thin blood–alveolar surface to maximize gaseous exchange. Gas exchange in the lung is limited by perfusion because a rise in blood flow increases the rate of oxygen uptake as it maintains the concentration gradient for oxygen uptake between the alveoli and the capillaries.

Pulmonary arteries and arterioles are shorter, have thinner walls and are more distensible than systemic vessels (they share many characteristics with venous vessels). This means that pulmonary vascular resistance is very low and pulmonary arterial pressures are much lower than systemic blood pressures (22/8 mmHg). Remember, because right and left ventricular cardiac output have

to be equal, the lower pressures in the pulmonary vessels must be due to a lower pulmonary vascular resistance (analogous to total peripheral resistance). These low pressures, maintain low capillary pressures, preventing filtration of fluid into the alveolar interstitium.

In the upright position, mean pulmonary arterial pressure at the apex of the lung is about 3 mmHg, at the base it is about 21 mmHg, and at the level of the heart the mean pressure is 15 mmHg. These values are due to the effect of gravity. At the lung base, high pressure causes the thin-walled vessels to distend and blood flow to increase, while at the apex, flow only occurs during systole. The ventilation–perfusion ratio (V/Q) governs the efficiency of oxygen transfer. In an ideal scenario, the V/Q would be 1, meaning that alveolar ventilation and alveolar perfusion are proportional in all parts of the lungs. Although ventilation is also greater at the bases than at the apex, the difference is not as great as the difference in perfusion (Fig. 5.18). This causes a V/Q >1 at the apex and a V/Q <1 at the bases. In the lungs as a whole, the V/Q is approximately 0.8.

One adaptation of the pulmonary circulation that aims to improve the V/Q is called hypoxic pulmonary vasoconstriction. In this process, vessels in poorly ventilated areas of the lung, in which pO_2 is low, undergo vasoconstriction to limit blood flow to that underventilated area. This mechanism helps to optimize ventilation–perfusion ratios. This response to hypoxia is a contrast to that in the systemic circulation in which hypoxia tends to bring about a vasodilatation.

Cutaneous circulation

The skin has a low metabolic requirement, and its vasculature is primarily involved in the regulation of the core body temperature. Specific areas of the skin have

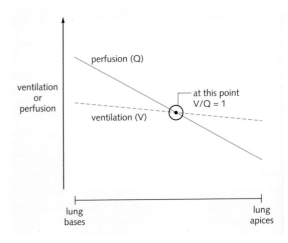

Fig. 5.18 The relationship between ventilation and perfusion in different areas of the lungs.

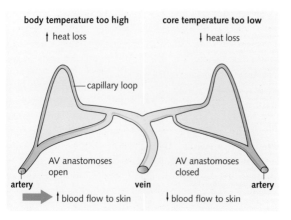

body temperature too high	core temperature too low
↑ heat loss	↓ heat loss

capillary loop

AV anastomoses open AV anastomoses closed

artery   vein   artery

↑ blood flow to skin   ↓ blood flow to skin

Fig. 5.19 Temperature control by arteriovenous (AV) anastomoses.

arteriovenous (AV) anastomoses (Fig. 5.19). These exposed areas have a high surface area to volume ratio and include the fingers, toes, palms, soles of the feet, lips, nose and ears. The VSM tone in these anastomoses is controlled by sympathetic vasoconstrictor nerves, the activity of which is determined by the brainstem. This sympathetic outflow from the brainstem is influenced by the temperature-regulating area in the hypothalamus. When temperature is low, sympathetic outflow to the skin is increased, constricting the AV anastamoses, diverting blood to the internal venous vessels and decreasing cutaneous perfusion. Skin temperature is very variable as it is influenced by ambient temperature. It has a direct effect on cutaneous vascular tone:

- Local heating causes vasodilatation, increasing cutaneous blood flow.

- Local cooling causes vasoconstriction, decreasing cutaneous blood flow.

Paradoxical cold vasodilatation occurs in the extremities on prolonged exposure to cold. After the initial vasoconstriction, vasodilatation occurs. This is thought to be because the cold impairs sympathetic vasoconstriction.

The cutaneous circulation is an important target of baroreceptor-mediated vasoconstriction in response to a reduction in blood pressure. This constriction is brought about by sympathetic nerves, circulating catecholamines, ADH and angiotensin II and is responsible for the cold, pale hands found in patients in shock. Emotion can produce a hyperaemic response in the skin (blushing) and the gastric and colonic mucosa. Compression of the skin for long periods (e.g. when sitting) impairs blood flow. Reactive hyperaemia and the skin's high tolerance to hypoxia prevent ischaemic damage.

In hot weather, cutaneous vasodilatation can reduce venous return. This can lead to fainting by virtue of decreased cardiac output and cerebral hypoperfusion. When soldiers stand on a hot day, they must use their skeletal muscle pumps to maintain venous return from their legs and prevent this happening.

HINTS AND TIPS

Raynaud's phenomenon is a condition whereby exposure of the extremities (fingers, toes, nose) causes an excessive cutaneous vasoconstriction that impairs perfusion of the extremities resulting in ischaemia.

Integrated control of the cardiovascular system and cardiovascular reflexes

6

● **Objectives**

You should be able to:

- Understand the function and importance of baroreceptors and the baroreceptor reflex.
- Describe the central pathways that influence the cardiovascular system.
- Describe the important cardiorespiratory reflexes and their importance.
- Understand the changes that take place during the Valsalva manoeuvre.
- Describe the cardiovascular causes of syncope.
- Understand the cardiovascular changes that occur during dynamic and static exercise.
- Describe the different types of shock and the compensatory changes that take place in response to haemorrhage.

ARTERIAL BARORECEPTORS AND THE BAROREFLEX

The baroreceptor reflex plays a key role in the minute-to-minute control of arterial blood pressure. Arterial baroreceptors are stretch receptors located in the wall of the carotid sinuses and the aortic arch. They continuously generate impulses, the frequency of which depends on the degree of vessel wall stretch. Increased stretch (due to increased pressure), also known as increased baroreceptor loading, increases firing rate, whereas decreased stretch (baroreceptor unloading) decreases the firing rate. The impulses generated by the baroreceptors are carried to the nucleus tractus solitarius (NTS) in the medulla by the glossopharyngeal (carotid sinus) and vagus nerves (aortic arch). In the NTS, these afferent impulses interact with other central pathways regulating autonomic nervous system activity.

When blood pressure decreases, the baroreceptors are unloaded (stretch is reduced) and the firing rate to the medulla decreases. The effect is to decrease parasympathetic (PNS) and increase sympathetic (SNS) drive. This results in:

- Increased heart rate and contractility, increasing cardiac output (SNS and PNS).
- Peripheral vasoconstriction, increasing total peripheral resistance (SNS).
- Venoconstriction, decreasing venous pooling and increasing venous return and preload (SNS).
- Catecholamine secretion (SNS).
- Increased renin secretion and activation of the renin–angiotensin system, causing vasoconstriction and increasing circulating volume (SNS).

These responses are illustrated in Fig. 6.1.

The effect is to increase cardiac output and total peripheral resistance, restoring blood pressure to its normal level. The baroreflex is very rapid and it is very important in acute hypotension and haemorrhage. The increase in renin secretion will lead to increased angiotensin II and aldosterone production, which will increase circulating volume. This effect, however, is much slower than the other four. Increased loading of the baroreceptors has the opposite effect, decreasing cardiac output and total peripheral resistance.

The vascular beds that are primarily affected by baroreceptor-mediated vasoconstriction are those in the skeletal muscle and the gastrointestinal tract. The cutaneous circulation is also important if the temperature is neutral. The cerebral and coronary circulations are largely unaffected by these changes in sympathetic activity.

The level of blood pressure that the baroreceptors take as 'normal' (the set point) can be reset by central or peripheral processes:

- Central resetting: in exercise or during 'fight or flight' situations, the rise in blood pressure that occurs does not cause a bradycardia because there are central influences that reset the baroreflex set point and allow the blood pressure to increase.
- Peripheral resetting: chronic hyper- or hypotension leads to the set point being reset to this new pressure, thus allowing the baroreflex to operate in its optimal range. For this reason, the baroreflex is not very useful for long-term blood pressure homeostasis.

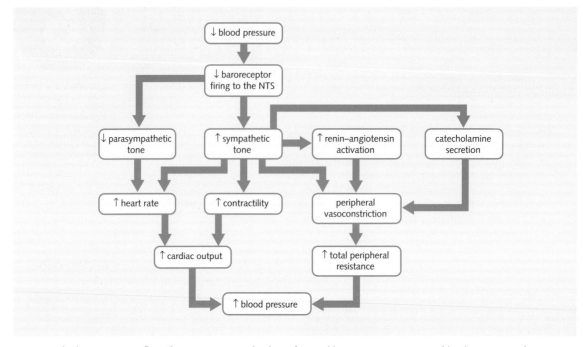

Fig. 6.1 The baroreceptor reflex. The responses to unloading of arterial baroreceptors to restore blood pressure to the set point (NTS, nucleus tractus solitarius).

The sensitivity of the arterial baroreceptors to a change in blood pressure is decreased by:

- Age: the compliance of the arterial wall falls with age, which means that the arterial walls require a greater increase in pressure in order to stretch them.
- Chronic hypertension: arteriosclerosis decreases arterial compliance.

Central pathways

The central pathways that influence the cardiovascular system involve a complex interaction between the medulla, hypothalamus and cortex.

Medulla

It used to be thought that there was a specific vasomotor centre in the medulla. Now, it is thought that there are complex signals between the hypothalamus, cortex and cerebellum as well as signals within the vasomotor centre of the medulla:

- The rostral ventrolateral medulla is responsible for the sympathetic outflow.
- The nucleus ambiguus is responsible for the parasympathetic (vagal) outflow.

Together, these two areas mediate the neural control of vascular tone and heart rate. Information from baroreceptors and other cardiovascular receptors is received at the nucleus tractus solitarius in the medulla. The afferent inputs are integrated and relayed to other areas in the brain.

Hypothalamus

The hypothalamus contains four areas of interest:

- Depressor area: this receives input from the NTS and can produce the baroreflex but is not vital for the reflex to occur.
- Defence area: this is responsible for the alerting or 'fight or flight' response, thus playing a role in governing sympathetic outflow.
- Temperature-regulating area: this controls cutaneous vascular tone and sweating to regulate body temperature.
- ADH-secreting area: this produces antidiuretic hormone (vasopressin), which travels through nerve axons to the posterior pituitary where it is released into the bloodstream.

CARDIORESPIRATORY INTERACTIONS

The first cardiorespiratory interaction is described in Chapter 4. During inspiration, the decrease in intrathoracic pressure increases venous return. This increases stroke volume by Starling's law. In addition to this mechanical interaction, there are also neurally mediated cardiorespiratory interactions.

Sinus arrhythmia (Fig. 6.2)

Sinus arrhythmia describes the increase in heart rate that occurs during inspiration and is a normal phenomenon. It is more profound in younger people and tends to subside with age. There are two mechanisms that underlie sinus arrhythmia:

1. The first is a CNS influence. The motor neurons that stimulate the inspiratory muscles have an inhibitory influence on the nucleus ambiguus. This decreases vagal activity to the heart, increasing heart rate.
2. The second is a reflex mediated process initiated by pulmonary stretch receptors in the airways. As inspiration proceeds and the chest expands, activity of these stretch receptors increases. This also has an inhibitory effect on the nucleus ambiguous (via the vagus nerve), again decreasing vagal drive and increasing heart rate.

In addition to producing sinus arrhythmia under resting conditions, these two mechanisms also underpin the increase in heart rate that occurs in any situation where respiratory rate is increased. Examples include systemic hypoxia, exercise and stress. The reverse is also true in that decreased respiratory rate leads to a decrease in heart rate.

Arterial chemoreceptors

Peripheral chemoreceptors are located in the carotid and aortic bodies. They are involved in the regulation of oxygen and carbon dioxide levels in arterial blood and the arterial blood pH. Their fibres travel with afferent baroreceptor fibres in the glossopharyngeal and vagus nerves. Their activity is increased by increased carbon dioxide, decreased oxygen and reduced pH in the arterial blood.

The primary cardiovascular reflex caused by increased stimulation of these chemoreceptors is an increase in parasympathetic drive to the heart, decreasing heart rate, and an increase in sympathetic drive to the arterioles, causing vasoconstriction. This reflex is in place to reduce oxygen requirements; however, it is only apparent if the respiratory rate is not able to increase, for example when a person is paralysed, being artificially ventilated or when a baby is in the mother's womb.

> **HINTS AND TIPS**
>
> In the fetus, a decrease in heart rate suggests that the fetus is hypoxic. It is this chemoreceptor reflex that underpins this phenomenon.

Under normal circumstances, when respiratory rate can increase, increased stimulation of the chemoreceptors increases outflow from the inspiratory centre, increasing respiratory rate and tidal volume. As is described above, this causes an increase in heart rate, and the greater degree of pulmonary stretch receptor stimulation that accompanies increased tidal volume will further augment this response. These responses

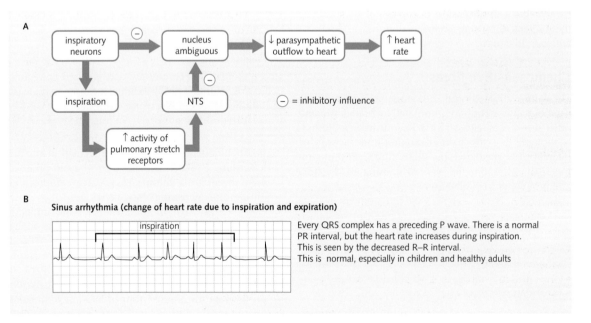

Fig. 6.2 (A) Neural pathways underpinning sinus arrhythmia and the increase in heart rate in response to an increased respiratory rate or increased tidal volume. (B) ECG trace of sinus arrhythmia (NTS, nucleus tractus solitarius).

are superimposed on the primary cardiovascular reflex and under normal circumstances, hypoxaemia (reduced oxygen in the blood) causes a tachycardia. Remember that hypoxaemia will also cause vasodilatation in certain vascular beds such as skeletal muscle and the brain via the local effects of reduced partial pressure of oxygen in the blood.

Other cardiopulmonary receptors

There are many cardiopulmonary receptors in the heart, great veins and pulmonary arteries with afferents to the NTS. There are three other classes of receptor not yet described, each with differing functions: atrial stretch receptors, unmyelinated mechanoreceptor fibres and chemosensitive fibres.

Atrial stretch receptors

These are branched nerve endings located where the great veins join the atria and are connected to large myelinated vagal fibres. They are stimulated by atrial stretch, which is increased when blood volume increases. Stimulation produces a reflex tachycardia (the Bainbridge reflex) by selectively increasing sympathetic drive to the sinoatrial node. It also decreases secretion of antidiuretic hormone promoting water excretion in order to reduce circulating volume.

Unmyelinated mechanoreceptor fibres

These are present in both atria and in the left ventricle. Afferent fibres travel in vagal and sympathetic nerves. Large degrees of distension in the chambers stimulate these receptors causing a reflex bradycardia and peripheral vasodilatation.

Chemosensitive fibres

These unmyelinated vagal and sympathetic afferents are chemosensitive. They are stimulated by bradykinin and other substances released by ischaemic myocardium. It is thought that the pain of angina and myocardial infarction is mediated by these fibres. Stimulation increases respiration as well as causing bradycardia and peripheral vasodilatation.

COORDINATED CARDIOVASCULAR RESPONSES

Orthostasis

When moving from a supine position to standing (orthostasis), the effect of gravity causes venous pooling in any vessels below the heart; thus venous pressures increase and the veins distend. This causes a fall in apparent circulation volume and venous return. Cardiac filling is reduced and stroke volume and cardiac output fall. Arterial blood pressure drops, but this hypotension is only transient as the baroreceptor reflex corrects it almost immediately. If there is already a degree of peripheral vasodilatation, due to high temperature for example, this transient hypotension may be enough to cause cerebral hypoperfusion and cause the person to faint.

Upon standing, the baroreceptors decrease their firing rate and cardiopulmonary receptors decrease their firing rate in response to reduced cardiac blood volume. This increases sympathetic outflow and decreases parasympathetic drive, resulting in an increased heart rate (of about 20 bpm) and contractility. Peripheral vasoconstriction increases total peripheral resistance, which helps restore the blood pressure. Venoconstriction also plays a role in helping to reverse venous pooling, particularly the splanchnic veins. Capillary filtration in the legs increases because of the increase in venous pressure, which may cause a reduction in plasma volume over time. Reduced activity in the baroreceptors and cardiopulmonary receptors also increases secretion of ADH and aldosterone (via renin–angiotensin), which promote salt and water retention in order to increase plasma volume. The overall effect is maintenance of arterial pressure and, thus, cerebral perfusion.

Failure of this mechanism causes postural hypotension, defined as a decrease in systolic blood pressure of >15 mmHg on standing which may be associated with symptoms of light-headedness or even collapse.

Valsalva manoeuvre

The Valsalva manoeuvre is a forced expiration against a closed glottis. This commonly occurs when coughing, defecating, or lifting heavy weights. It causes an increase in intrathoracic pressure, which brings about a cardiovascular response that proceeds in four stages (Fig. 6.3).

- Stage 1: the increase in intrathoracic pressure increases flow of blood from the pulmonary circulation into the left atrium. This increases left ventricular end-diastolic volume and stroke volume. There is also compression of the aorta, increasing blood pressure.
- Stage 2: the high intrathoracic pressure impedes venous return and the resulting reduction in filling pressures decreases stroke volume and thus blood pressure. During this period, there is a baroreceptor-mediated increase in heart rate.
- Stage 3: when the manoeuvre is released, the compression on the aorta is stopped and left ventricular filling pressures are reduced temporarily as the pulmonary vessels re-expand. This causes a drop in blood pressure.

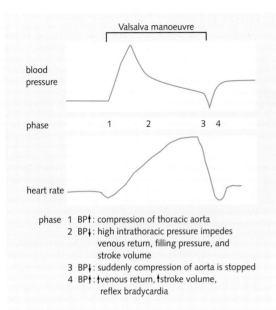

Fig. 6.3 Response to the Valsalva manoeuvre (BP, blood pressure).

phase 1 BP↑: compression of thoracic aorta
2 BP↓: high intrathoracic pressure impedes venous return, filling pressure, and stroke volume
3 BP↓: suddenly compression of aorta is stopped
4 BP↑: ↑venous return, ↑stroke volume, reflex bradycardia

- Stage 4: venous return is restored, increasing cardiac filling pressures and stroke volume. This increases blood pressure and a baroreceptor reflex-mediated bradycardia.

This manoeuvre is a useful test of baroreceptor competence. If the pressure fall in phase 2 continues and there is no bradycardia in phase 4, then the baroreflex is interrupted, and the person will be at risk of postural hypotension.

Diving reflex

The diving reflex occurs when cold water stimulates the sensory receptors of the trigeminal nerve on the face, and receptors in the nasopharynx and oropharynx. The body is expecting a dive into water and a period of submersion. The response is in place to conserve the limited oxygen supply available during submersion and to preferentially divert it to the heart and brain. The reflex results in three changes:

- Apnoea (no breathing): while apnoeic, the changing concentrations of oxygen and carbon dioxide in the blood will stimulate the chemoreceptors, decreasing heart rate by increasing vagal drive.
- Bradycardia: caused by intense vagal inhibition of the pacemaker potential, decreases oxygen consumption.
- Peripheral vasoconstriction: occurs in the splanchnic, renal and skeletal muscle vascular beds. The strong, sympathetically mediated vasoconstriction overwhelms any metabolic dilatation that may occur in active muscle and the increase in total peripheral

resistance allows blood pressure to be maintained despite the profound bradycardia.

The alerting/defence response

This is the body's response to a stressful stimulus. This may be pain, a frightening noise, a stressful situation or in anticipation of exercise. It is also known as the 'fight or flight' response. The components of the response are as follows:

- There is an increase in sympathetic outflow and decrease in parasympathetic outflow to the heart. This increases heart rate and contractility, increasing cardiac output.
- Increased sympathetic outflow to the gastrointestinal tract (GIT), kidneys and skin causes vasoconstriction.
- Decreased sympathetic outflow to skeletal muscle reduces arteriolar tone causing vasodilatation.
- Release of adrenaline/epinephrine from the adrenal medulla further increases heart rate and contractility by binding myocardial β_1 receptors. It also acts on α_1 receptors causing vasoconstriction in the skin and gut, and β_2 receptors in skeletal muscle causing vasodilatation.

The net result is an increase in heart rate and blood pressure, and an increase in skeletal muscle blood flow. It is important to remember that during this response the baroreceptor reflex is inhibited so the increase in blood pressure is not corrected. The changes in autonomic activity also cause pupillary dilatation and piloerection. The degree to which these changes take place is graded by the intensity of the stimulus and the intensity of the response. The responses of two different people to the same stimulus may be very different.

Syncope (fainting)

Syncope is a sudden, transient loss of consciousness as a result of impaired cerebral perfusion. It may be initiated by orthostasis, severe hypovolaemia, arrhythmia or by psychological stress (e.g. fear, pain or horror). In psychogenic syncope, there is often a pre-syncope period of tachycardia, cutaneous vasoconstriction, hyperventilation and sweating, produced by the alerting response described above. During this period, hyperventilation causes a reduction in the concentration of carbon dioxide in the blood and can cause paraesthesia in the fingers and around the mouth. This prodrome is followed by the vasovagal episode that produces loss of consciousness.

A vasovagal episode proceeds as follows:

1. A sudden large increase in vagal outflow causes a bradycardia.
2. Profound peripheral vasodilatation occurs due to decreased sympathetic drive.
3. This causes a fall in blood pressure, reducing cerebral blood flow.
4. If it occurs at all, loss of consciousness results within seconds.

> **HINTS AND TIPS**
>
> Fits, faints and funny turns are very common presentations of cardiovascular disease. It is important to consider a number of pathologies in the nervous, cardiovascular and respiratory systems before reaching the diagnosis of a psychological cause. A thorough history and an open mind will help prevent you from making mistakes!

The cause of the sudden changes is unknown. In psychogenic fainting, it could be a primitive 'playing dead' response. In hypovolaemic syncope and arrhythmia, it could be triggered by activity of ventricular mechanoreceptors, which are strongly activated by contraction of the near-empty left ventricle.

A person who has fainted falls to the floor and ends up in the supine position. This raises the intrathoracic blood volume and the cardiac filling pressures, and lowers the head to the same level as the heart. Coupled with the baroreflex, this then increases cardiac output and arterial pressure, restoring cerebral perfusion. Consciousness is restored in under 2 minutes. You should never hold a person who has fainted upright as this prevents the beneficial effects of increasing intrathoracic blood volume and may maintain cerebral hypoperfusion. Raising the person's legs will cause a further increase in venous return and thus cardiac output.

Cardiovascular response to exercise

During exercise, there are a number of cardiovascular responses in place to increase blood flow to the active muscles while maintaining a stable blood pressure.

Initial requirements during exercise are:

- Increased gaseous exchange in the pulmonary circulation.
- Increased blood flow to the working muscle and decreasing blood flow to inactive muscle and other tissues.
- Maintenance of stable blood pressure.

Dynamic exercise

During dynamic exercise (e.g. walking, running or cycling), there is increased production of vasodilator metabolites in the active muscles that stimulate a metabolic hyperaemia. This vasodilatation increases delivery of oxygen and nutrients to the active muscle, but were it to occur in isolation, it would reduce total peripheral resistance and decrease the blood pressure. The exercise reflex is superimposed on the locally mediated functional hyperaemia and is in place to allow all of the above requirements to be satisfied simultaneously.

The exercise reflex is stimulated by afferent inputs from metaboreceptors in active muscle, which increase their activity in response to metabolites of cellular respiration, and joint receptors activated by joint movement. These signals travel to the hypothalamic locomotor area in the brain, which initiates the cardiorespiratory changes that comprise the exercise reflex. These include:

- Increased sympathetic and decreased parasympathetic outflow to the heart increasing heart rate and increasing contractility. This increases cardiac output, increasing pulmonary blood flow and oxygenation as well as increasing tissue perfusion.
- Increased respiratory rate. This increases oxygenation in the pulmonary vasculature and also further decreases vagal outflow to the heart, increasing heart rate.
- Increased sympathetic outflow to the vessels of the skeletal muscle, GIT, spleen, kidneys and cutaneous circulation brings about vasoconstriction. The increased sympathetic outflow to the active muscles, however, is overcome by the local metabolic hyperaemia. The vasoconstriction in the skin persists until there is an increase in core body temperature, at which time the cutaneous vessels dilate in order to regulate the body temperature. Sympathetic venoconstriction (particularly in the spleen) also occurs, increasing venous return.
- Increased levels of circulating catecholamines cause selective vasodilatation in skeletal muscle while constricting other beds. This also increases cardiac output.

There are also a number of passive changes that occur during dynamic exercise:

- The skeletal muscle pump decreases venous pressure in the active muscles, increasing the perfusion pressure of the muscle. The skeletal pump also increases venous return and thus stroke volume.

- In addition to increasing blood flow, the metabolic vasodilatation increases the proportion of capillary units that are being perfused, increasing the surface area available for exchange of metabolic substrates in the active muscles.

Static exercise

During static exercise, the prolonged skeletal muscle contraction compresses the blood vessels within the active muscle, increasing the resistance to flow. This is a similar idea to that in the coronary arteries when blood flow occurs during diastole rather than systole when the vessels are compressed. This effect prevents the increase in muscle blood flow that is stimulated by local production of metabolites. The vascular smooth muscle in the arterioles does relax but the extrinsic compression of the vessels keeps them occluded. In the absence of increased blood flow to the contracting muscle, the levels of metabolites in the muscle rise further, increasing stimulation of muscle metaboreceptors, bringing about an exaggerated exercise reflex (as described above) compared with that seen during dynamic exercise. When

contraction is released, and the vessels are no longer compressed, there is a profound vasodilatation and blood flow to the muscles increases significantly.

Blood pressure during static and dynamic exercise (Fig. 6.4)

During dynamic exercise the mean arterial blood pressure remains fairly stable and may increase slightly. The increase in cardiac output and sympathetically mediated vasoconstriction stimulated by the exercise reflex act to increase blood pressure (and do increase systolic pressure) while the metabolic vasodilatation in active muscles and the cutaneous vasodilatation in place to regulate body temperature decrease total peripheral resistance and decrease diastolic pressure. The increased systolic and decreased diastolic pressure result in a relatively small change in mean pressure and a marked increase in pulse pressure.

During static exercise, the systolic blood pressure increases as a result of the exercise reflex but the compression of vessels in the active muscles prevents the decrease

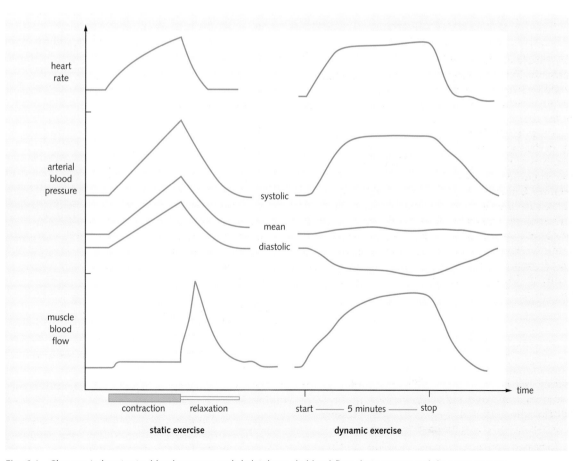

Fig. 6.4   Changes in heart rate, blood pressure and skeletal muscle blood flow during static and dynamic exercise.

in total peripheral resistance and in fact increases resistance, increasing diastolic blood pressure. The increases in both SBP and DBP increase mean arterial pressure significantly.

Anaerobic exercise

During aerobic exercise, the metabolic vasodilatation in active muscle combined with the exercise reflex maintains adequate oxygen delivery to the active muscle. During anaerobic exercise, which is defined as when the cardiovascular response is inadequate to meet the demands of the active tissues, carbon dioxide and lactate production are increased. This causes a decrease in blood pH, which stimulates the arterial chemoreceptors. As described above, increased chemoreceptor stimulation leads to an increase in respiratory rate and tidal volume, increasing alveolar ventilation. This brings about an increase in ventilation in excess of that required to maintain oxygen, allowing more carbon dioxide to be blown off, decreasing the arterial P_{CO_2} and correcting the arterial pH.

SHOCK AND HAEMORRHAGE

Haemorrhage

Haemorrhage describes loss of blood from the vascular compartment and can occur either externally from an open wound or internally (into the abdominal or thoracic compartment, for example). The body has a number of responses in place in order to initially to compensate for the reduction in circulating volume and eventually to replace that volume. Acute haemorrhage can be classified according to the amount of blood lost or the percentage of total blood volume lost. Fig. 6.5 shows this classification and the changes in physiological parameters that occur at each stage.

In the absence of compensatory cardiovascular changes, haemorrhage will reduce circulating volume and reduce blood pressure by virtue of Starling's law decreasing stroke volume. The reduction in blood pressure would be dependent on the amount of blood lost as that would determine the degree to which ventricular filling (preload) was reduced. In reality, however, changes do take place and these can be divided into three sets based on the timeframe in which they occur (Fig. 6.6):

Immediate response (seconds to minutes)

The immediate response is a baroreceptor-mediated response stimulated by the decrease in blood pressure. The increased sympathetic outflow and decrease in renal perfusion stimulate the release of renin and thus production of angiotensin II and ADH. Levels of circulating adrenaline/epinephrine and noradrenaline/norepinephrine also increase. All of these hormones exert an additional vasoconstrictor effect, supporting the baroreceptor-mediated response. The decrease in stroke volume and the increase in total peripheral resistance may maintain mean blood pressure but is likely to reduce the pulse pressure (remember SV influences SBP and TPR influences DBP). It is important to remember that in this immediate response, the changes simply aim to maintain blood pressure and perfusion of the brain and the heart; they in no way correct the loss of circulating volume. The intense arteriolar vasoconstriction can (if severe enough) impair perfusion of peripheral tissues and cause a metabolic acidosis (due to increased lactate production). This will inevitably happen if the loss of circulating volume is not corrected and will stimulate the arterial chemoreceptors, increasing respiratory rate.

Fig. 6.5 Changes in vital signs in response to acute haemorrhage

Parameter	Class I	Class II	Class III	Class IV
Blood loss (%)	0–15	15–30	30–40	>40
Blood loss (mL)	0–750	750–1500	1500–2000	>2000
Pulse rate	↔	↑	↑	↑↑
Respiratory rate	↔	↑	↑↑	↑↑
Capillary refill time	↔	↔	↑	↑↑
Blood pressure	↔	↔	Narrowing of pulse pressure	↓

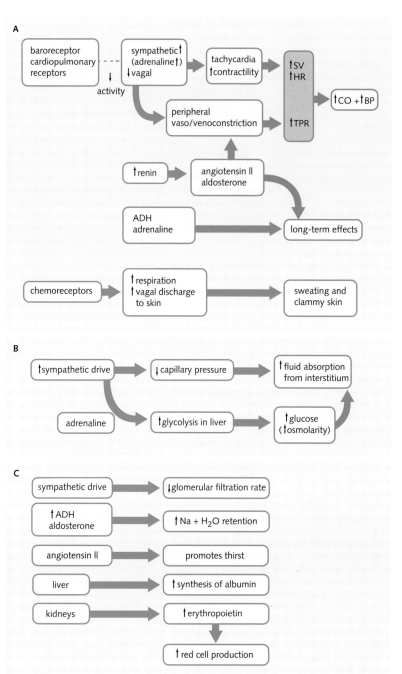

Fig. 6.6 (A) Immediate response to haemorrhage (ADH, antidiuretic hormone; BP, blood pressure; CO, cardiac output; HR, heart rate; SV, stroke volume; TPR, total peripheral resistance). (B) Intermediate response to haemorrhage. (C) Long-term response to haemorrhage (ADH, antidiuretic hormone).

Intermediate response (minutes to hours)

The profound vasoconstriction and venoconstriction described above decreases the capillary hydrostatic pressure at both the arteriolar and the venous end of the capillaries. This will decrease the capillary hydrostatic pressure and bring about increased fluid absorption from the interstitial compartment. This effect can be augmented by a small increase in plasma osmolality caused by increased glucose concentration due to adrenaline/epinephrine stimulating hepatic glycolysis, which increases capillary oncotic pressure. This movement of fluid from the interstitium to the vascular compartment can be described as an autotransfusion. This autotransfusion response is not a compensatory change but rather acts to correct the loss of circulating volume, but is unlikely to do so completely.

Long-term response (hours to days)

The activation of the renin–angiotensin system and increased levels of ADH and aldosterone all stimulate sodium and water retention in the renal tubules, increasing plasma volume. Angiotensin II stimulates thirst, increasing water intake if the patient is able to do so. Although these responses increase circulating volume (given time), they do so with water, and do not replace the red blood cells, clotting factors, plasma proteins and other humoral components of blood that were lost. This causes a dilutional reduction in haemoglobin, which is corrected by increased release of erythropoietin (stimulates red blood cell production in the bone marrow) from the kidney.

> Think about what happens to the blood haemoglobin (Hb) concentration during haemorrhage and the subsequent compensatory changes. Initially, when blood is lost, the Hb concentration will stay the same (although the total amount is reduced). The autotransfusion will then decrease the concentration of Hb by a small degree by diluting it slightly. As plasma volume is restored, by IV fluids, oral fluids or reabsorption in the kidneys, Hb will continue to be diluted, causing the concentration to decrease further. Erythropoietin production will increase red blood cell production (and thus Hb concentration) but this effect is much slower than the volume restoration.

The primary aims in the treatment of haemorrhage are firstly, to stop the bleeding and secondly, to replace circulating volume with intravenous fluids as appropriate. It is important to remember that replacement does not have to be with blood; the key is to restore circulating volume to ensure cardiac output is sufficient to maintain perfusion of the vital organs.

Shock

Shock is an acute failure of the cardiovascular system to adequately perfuse the tissues of the body. Shock can be divided in to four categories depending upon the causative factor:

- Hypovolaemic shock.
- Cardiogenic shock.
- Obstructive shock.
- Septic shock.

Shock (except septic shock, dealt with separately) causes a characteristic clinical picture, the components of which can all be predicted with a knowledge of the compensatory changes that occur in response to a decrease in cardiac output and blood pressure. They can include the following:

- Pale, cold, clammy skin caused by cutaneous vasoconstriction in an effort to maintain adequate blood flow to the vital organs.
- Sweating caused by sympathetic stimulation.
- Rapid, weak pulse caused by compensatory tachycardia and decreased stroke volume.
- Reduced pulse pressure due to reduced stroke volume (reduced SBP) and increased total peripheral resistance (increased DBP).
- Rapid, shallow breathing as a result of chemoreceptor stimulation by reduced blood pH from metabolic acidosis caused by anaerobic cellular respiration (in the presence of inadequate oxygen delivery).
- Reduced urine output due to renal hypoperfusion and reduced glomerular filtration.

Hypovolaemic shock

This results from a fall in circulating blood volume caused by either:

- external fluid loss (e.g. vomiting, diarrhoea, haemorrhage), or
- internal fluid loss (e.g. pancreatitis, internal bleeding).

Cardiogenic shock

This is caused by an impairment of cardiac function such that the heart is unable to maintain adequate cardiac output, i.e. pump failure. It usually has an acute onset, but it may be a result of worsening heart failure. Causes include:

- Myocardial infarction.
- Arrhythmia.
- Severe heart failure.

Obstructive shock

In obstructive shock there is a direct obstruction to blood entering or leaving the heart or great vessels, for example:

- Cardiac tamponade (discussed in Ch. 8).
- Massive pulmonary embolism: this restricts pulmonary blood flow, preventing blood from reaching the left side of the heart, impairing left ventricular filling and limiting preload.

Septic shock

Sepsis is caused by toxins (e.g. endotoxin) released from certain bacteria during infection. This initiates a profound systemic inflammatory response, with production of cytokines and inflammatory mediators. This causes a widespread vasodilatation and an increase in capillary permeability. Total peripheral resistance falls and leakage of plasma proteins into the interstitial fluid causes movement of fluid from the vascular compartment into the interstitium, decreasing circulating volume. This reduces circulating volume, decreasing venous return and stroke volume, which, combined with the decrease in total peripheral resistance, significantly decreases blood pressure. Although the baroreceptor reflex causes a tachycardia and increases myocardial contractility, increasing cardiac output, the peripheral vasoconstriction is ineffective. The patient will have a tachycardia but warm skin and a low blood pressure due to the widespread vasodilatation. Treatment is with fluid replacement, antibiotics and, if severe, can include noradrenaline/norepinephrine to bring about vasoconstriction and restore blood pressure.

Anaphylaxis

Anaphylaxis is a rapidly developing, life threatening, severe, type I hypersensitivity reaction. It is an immediate IgE-mediated immune response to an antigen in the body to which the patient is 'allergic'. It leads to rapid circulatory collapse (shock), dyspnoea, and potentially death. The IgE immune response consists of the activation of basophils and mast cells, leading to release of histamine and other factors. Prostaglandins, leukotrienes, thromboxane, and platelet activation factors are also synthesized and released. The results are as follows:

- Generalized peripheral vasodilatation.
- Increased vascular permeability causes leakage of plasma protein into the interstitium increasing tissue oncotic pressure, causing movement of fluid into the interstitium and reducing plasma volume.
- Bronchial smooth muscle constriction, restricting ventilation.
- Oral, laryngeal, and pharyngeal oedema, which may compromise the airway.
- Urticaria and flushing.

The most important step in the treatment of anaphylaxis is administration of intramuscular adrenaline/epinephrine. This reverses the bronchoconstriction by acting on β_2 receptors and increases blood pressure by increasing cardiac output via action on β_1 receptors and vasoconstriction via action on α_1 receptors. Administration of antihistamine (e.g. chlorphenamine) and IV hydrocortisone dampen the immune response.

Atherosclerosis and ischaemic heart disease

7

You should be able to:

- Understand the pathological basis of arteriosclerosis and atherosclerosis.
- List the modifiable and non-modifiable risk factors for atherosclerosis and ischaemic heart disease.
- Understand the principle of primary and secondary prevention and its application in ischaemic heart disease.
- Describe how lipids are transported and metabolized and how this is modified with drugs.
- Understand the basis of stable angina and the investigations available for its assessment.
- Describe the treatment options for stable angina and the rationale for their use.
- Understand the process of platelet activation and thrombus formation.
- Understand the classification of acute coronary syndromes and the pathological features of each.
- Describe the investigations for acute coronary syndromes and the rationale for their use.
- Understand the treatment options for acute coronary syndromes and the rationale for their use, in particular, antiplatelet and thrombolytic agents.

ARTERIOSCLEROSIS AND ATHEROSCLEROSIS

Arteriosclerosis

Arteriosclerosis is a term used to describe thickening and loss of elasticity of the arteries. Vessel thickening reduces lumen diameter, which may compromise organ perfusion. The loss of elasticity increases the likelihood of vessel rupture if exposed to increased mechanical stress. There are two important types of arteriosclerosis:

- Arteriolosclerosis: thickening of the wall in small arteries and arterioles, causes a reduction in lumen size. Often related to systemic hypertension and diabetes mellitus.
- Atherosclerosis: see below.

Atherosclerosis

Atherosclerosis is a progressive, inflammatory disease of large and medium sized arteries. It is characterized by focal accumulation of lipid in the vessel intima with an associated inflammatory and smooth muscle infiltrate. It is thought that atherosclerosis is present to some degree in all adults, and the consequences of atherosclerosis, which include ischaemic heart disease, peripheral vascular disease and cerebrovascular disease, are estimated to account for around 50% of deaths in Western societies.

Risk factors

Risk factors for atherosclerosis, and therefore risk factors for its associated conditions, can be broken down into 'modifiable' and 'non-modifiable', as follows:

Non-modifiable

- Age: increased age increases the number and severity of lesions.
- Sex: men are affected to a much greater extent than women, until the menopause when the incidence in women increases. This is thought to be due to the protective effects of oestrogens before menopause.
- Genetic predisposition: a family history of atherosclerotic disease increases an individual's risk significantly.

Modifiable

- Smoking.
- Hypertension.
- Diabetes mellitus.
- Hyperlipidaemia: high levels of low-density lipoprotein (LDL) cholesterol promote atherosclerosis while high-density lipoprotein (HDL) appears to be protective.

Other, less important factors involved in the development of atherosclerosis include a sedentary lifestyle, a diet high in saturated fat, and obesity.

Pathogenesis

The pathogenesis of atherosclerosis is often described by the response to injury hypothesis. This states that chronic damage to the vascular endothelium and the associated endothelial dysfunction are the key events in initiating the process. The steps involved in development of atherosclerosis are shown in Fig. 7.1 and include:

1. **Endothelial dysfunction:** chronic endothelial cell injury can occur as a result of cigarette smoking and high levels of cholesterol (particularly LDL), leading to metabolic dysfunction and structural changes. Damage activates endothelial cells, upregulating inflammatory adhesion molecules (e.g. ICAM-1) and promoting monocyte and platelet adhesion. This upregulation is also caused by altered gene expression at sites where the pattern of blood flow is altered, such as bends and bifurcation in vessels. Injury increases permeability to lipids and LDL, allowing their accumulation in the intima.

2. **Formation of a fatty streak:** monocytes adhere to the endothelium, migrate into the intima and differentiate into macrophages. Local oxidation of LDL is chemotactic for macrophages (attracts macrophages) and once in the intima, macrophages take up the oxidized LDL and become foam cells. Platelets adhere to activated endothelial cells or areas of denuded matrix and become activated. Activated platelets, activated endothelial cells and macrophages release platelet-derived growth factor (PDGF) stimulating smooth muscle cell migration from the media to the intima.

3. **Development of lipid plaque:** smooth muscle proliferation and an increase in extracellular matrix occur in the intima. Additional cytokines and growth factors produced by activated macrophages and platelets promote additional monocyte and smooth muscle infiltration. Lipid may also be released from dying foam cells, contributing to extracellular free lipid pools.

4. **Advanced plaques:** an advanced atherosclerotic plaque consists of a lipid rich 'core' and a fibrous 'cap'. The core of the lesion (which can become necrotic) consists of free lipid, macrophages, smooth muscle cells and cellular debris. The fibrous cap is composed primarily of collagen and lies over the core, beneath the endothelium.

A stable advanced atherosclerotic plaque, such as that depicted above, is likely to remain asymptomatic for years. Initially, as the plaque expands it causes remodelling of the media allowing the vessel to increase its diameter, accommodating the plaque without compromising the vessel lumen. This is the principle of Glagovian remodelling and the degree to which it occurs varies greatly. In the absence of this remodelling the plaque will grow, protruding into the lumen and progressively decreasing lumen size. It may only become apparent when the luminal diameter is not sufficient to allow adequate organ perfusion.

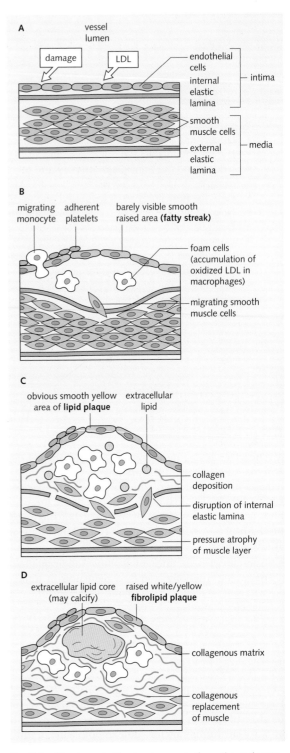

Fig. 7.1 The stages in the development of an atherosclerotic plaque, from the initial endothelial damage through to an advanced plaque. (A) Endothelial dysfunction. (B) Formation of the fatty streak. (C) Development of a lipid plaque. (D) Advanced atherosclerotic plaque (LDL, low-density lipoprotein).

The stability of the plaque is dependent on the strength and thickness of the fibrous cap, which relies on the balance between inflammation and repair. If this balance is disturbed and inflammation predominates, the cap may become thinner, less stable and may rupture. Atherosclerotic plaques also predispose to aneurysm formation (see Ch. 9).

LIPIDS AND THE CARDIOVASCULAR SYSTEM

Lipid transport and metabolism

The insolubility of lipids in plasma means a special transport mechanism is required. This is provided by lipid–protein complexes known as lipoproteins. The apolipoproteins (protein component of lipoproteins) also act as receptors for cell surface proteins, which determine the destination of different lipoproteins. Low-density lipoprotein (LDL) is the main lipoprotein involved in the transport of cholesterol. Fig. 7.2 shows the main transport pathways for lipids from the diet (exogenous) and for lipids from the body's stores (endogenous).

It is thought that apolipoprotein A is a prothrombotic lipoprotein that is particularly involved in coronary artery disease, while high levels of high-density lipoprotein (HDL) are protective. The classification of lipoproteins is outlined in Fig. 7.3.

Hyperlipidaemia

Hyperlipidaemia can be classified as hypertriglyceridaemia (raised triglycerides), hypercholesterolaemia (raised cholesterol), or hyperlipoproteinaemia (raised lipoproteins). In reality there may be combinations of each. Although these classifications are useful, they must be used with care because although hypercholesterolaemia is a risk factor for development of atherosclerosis, it is becoming increasingly apparent that the balance between LDL (damaging) and HDL (protective) may be more important than the absolute levels. As a result, some people prefer the term 'dyslipidaemia', as it refers to derangement of lipids rather than simply an increase.

HINTS AND TIPS

In patients with high cholesterol, lipids can be deposited in the subcutaneous tissues. Common sites include the skin around the eyes (xanthelasmas) and in tendons (tendon xanthomatas).

Treatment of hyperlipidaemia

Hyperlipidaemia can be treated with lifestyle interventions such as dietary changes or pharmacologically with drugs. Lifestyle interventions should include reduction of calorific intake, saturated fats and dietary cholesterol. Reduction of alcohol consumption and regular exercise are also beneficial. Supplements of omega-3 fats (present in fish oils) can be given as these may increase HDL levels.

There is no universally accepted level at which drug therapy should be started and the decision is usually based on assessment of overall risk of cardiovascular disease. NICE recommends treatment in primary prevention for anyone with a 10-year risk of greater than 20%. However, if cholesterol levels exceed 6 mmol/L, it will usually prompt treatment as a pathological disease in itself regardless of overall risk.

Drugs used to lower cholesterol

Statins (e.g. simvastatin, atorvastatin)

Statins are β-hydroxy-β-methylglutaryl coenzyme A HMG CoA reductase inhibitors. HMG CoA reductase is the rate-limiting step in cholesterol synthesis. When inhibited, the liver compensates for the decreased cholesterol synthesis by increasing LDL receptor expression, which decreases plasma levels of LDL. Statins are the first line drug for high cholesterol, can reduce cholesterol by more than 50%, and have been repeatedly demonstrated to reduce mortality in both primary and secondary prevention of cardiovascular disease. In addition to their cholesterol lowering effects, statins have an anti-atherosclerotic effect, reducing the inflammatory activity within atherosclerotic plaques (and thus strengthening the fibrous cap) and reducing the size of plaques. The main side-effects include reversible myositis and disturbed liver function tests.

Bile acid binding resins (e.g. colestipol and colestyramine)

Cholesterol is the initial substrate for synthesis of bile acids. These drugs bind bile acids in the intestine, forming insoluble complexes, increasing excretion of bile acids. In order to replenish bile acid levels, cholesterol is utilized for bile acid synthesis, thus reducing plasma cholesterol levels. This removes LDL cholesterol from circulation; however, these drugs can aggravate hypertriglyceridaemia.

Ezetimibe

This is a novel, orally acting selective inhibitor of cholesterol absorption. It may be used alone, or in combination with a statin in refractory cases. Despite its efficacy in lowering cholesterol (although only by about 10%), its benefit in terms of reducing mortality has been questioned.

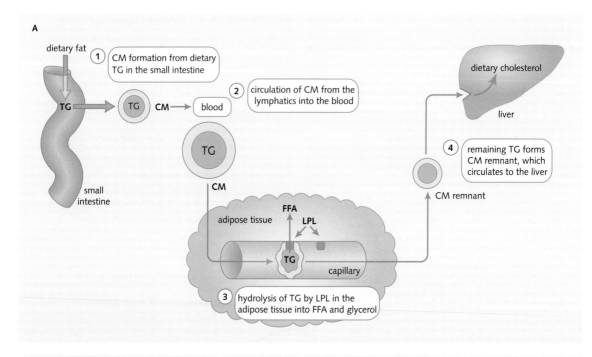

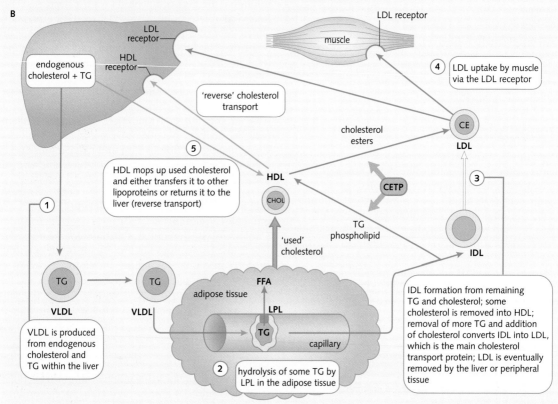

Fig. 7.2 (A) Exogenous and (B) endogenous lipid transport pathways (CE, cholesterol esters; CETP, cholesterol ester transfer protein; CM, chylomicron; FFA, free fatty acid; HDL, high-density lipoprotein; IDL, intermediate-density lipoprotein; LDL, low-density lipoprotein; LPL, lipoprotein lipase; TG, triacylglycerol; VLDL, very low-density lipoprotein).

Fig. 7.3 Classification of lipoproteins

Particle	Source	Predominantly transports
Chylomicron (CM)	Gut	Triacylglycerol
Very low-density lipoprotein (VLDL)	Liver	Triacylglycerol
Intermediate-density lipoprotein (IDL)	Catabolism	Cholesterol
Low-density lipoprotein (LDL)	Catabolism	Cholesterol
High-density lipoprotein (HDL)	Catabolism	Cholesterol
Lipoprotein A	Liver, gut	—

Fig. 7.4 Modifiable and non-modifiable risk factors for ischaemic heart disease

Non-modifiable	Modifiable
Sex (male) Age Family history Previous personal history	Smoking Diabetes Hypertension Hypercholesterolaemia Excessive alcohol Physical inactivity and obesity Stress

The main risk factors for ischaemic heart disease are the same as those for the development of atherosclerosis and are summarized again in Fig. 7.4.

HINTS AND TIPS

Knowledge of the risk factors for ischaemic heart disease is absolutely essential, both for examinations and for clinical practice.

Drugs used to lower triglyceride levels

Niacin
Niacin inhibits breakdown of fat in adipose tissue. This decreases plasma levels of free fatty acid, decreasing very low-density lipoprotein (VLDL) synthesis by the liver and, as a result, levels of intermediate-density lipoprotein (IDL) and LDL.

Fibrates
Gemfibrozil reduces lipolysis of triglycerides in adipose tissue, leading to decreased hepatic production of VLDL. Bezafibrate causes decreased VLDL and decreased triglycerides, but it may increase LDL. Fibrates are used mainly in familial hyperlipidaemia. Gemfibrozil is the better drug as it does not increase LDL.

Other, less common causes of myocardial ischaemia include the following:
- Coronary vasospasm: Prinzmetal's angina.
- Emboli as a result of infective endocarditis, or other causes such as thromboembolism.
- Vasculitis (e.g. polyarteritis nodosa, Kawasaki's syndrome).
- Shock: inadequate perfusion pressure.
- Severe aortic valvular disease: reduced coronary artery perfusion.
- Severe anaemia: reduced blood oxygen capacity.

ISCHAEMIC HEART DISEASE

Ischaemic heart disease (also called coronary heart disease) is the leading cause of death in the Western world and a great burden on the healthcare system. It is primarily a result of atherosclerosis in the coronary arteries.

Myocardial ischaemia occurs when the oxygen demand of the myocardium is greater than the supply of oxygen. Myocardial ischaemia can be caused by any or a combination of the following:

- Reduced blood supply to the myocardium, e.g. narrowing of coronary arteries.
- Increased demand of the myocardium, e.g. cardiac hypertrophy.
- Decreased oxygen content of blood reaching the myocardium, e.g. severe anaemia.

Risk prediction and primary prevention

Primary prevention aims to reduce a person's risk of developing ischaemic heart disease in the future. It involves treating seemingly healthy individuals, many of whom may never have developed the disease anyway. In order to guide doctors as to who will benefit most from primary prevention measures, various risk stratification models have been developed that estimate a person's risk of developing cardiovascular risk. The most widely used of these is the Framingham risk prediction chart and a sample of this is shown in Fig. 7.5. For those who are at high risk, lifestyle interventions and pharmacological measures are directed at reducing risk factors such as hypertension, hypercholesterolaemia (with a statin) and obesity.

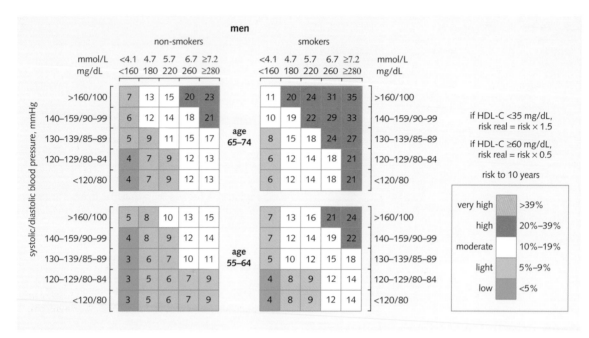

Fig. 7.5 A sample of the Framingham charts for estimating a patient's risk of cardiovascular disease. They take into account many of the major risk factors for cardiovascular disease and can be used to guide doctors when making decisions about medications for primary prevention.

Classification

The classification of ischaemic heart disease has changed in recent years and includes:

- Stable angina.
- Acute coronary syndromes (ACS): these include unstable angina and myocardial infarction, with or without ST elevation (STEMI and NSTEMI, respectively).

Stable angina

Angina is largely a clinical diagnosis, based on a history of 'heavy' or 'gripping' chest pain, typically in the centre, which may radiate to the arm, neck or jaw. Pain is usually provoked by physical exertion and subsides after a few minutes of rest. It can be worse on cold days or after a meal and is often accompanied by breathlessness. In most cases, angina is due to a stable atherosclerotic plaque in one or more coronary arteries causing a narrowing or stenosis (Fig. 7.6), but can result from coronary artery spasm (Prinzmetal's angina). On exertion, when myocardial oxygen demand is increased, the stenosed vessel prevents the necessary increase in blood flow, causing ischaemia and chest pain. At rest, when demand is lower, blood supply is adequate and symptoms subside. As a rule of thumb, it is said that the stenosis should reduce cross-sectional area of the vessel lumen by 70% in order to produce symptoms.

The following investigations can be performed in a patient with angina:

- Resting electrocardiogram (ECG): usually normal between episodes. During an attack, there may be ST segment depression and inverted T waves.
- Exercise ECG: useful for confirming the diagnosis and determining the extent of coronary artery disease. Patients have a continuous ECG trace recorded while undergoing a standardized exercise protocol on a treadmill (the Bruce protocol) until myocardial ischaemia is provoked, determined by ST depression >1 mm or chest pain.
- Myocardial perfusion scanning: this relies on the principle that when the myocardium is stressed (either by exercise or pharmacologically with a positive inotrope such as dobutamine), uptake of a radionucleotide tracer will be increased in line with the increase in perfusion. As a result, areas of myocardium which have impaired perfusion (due to stenosis in the arteries supplying them) will not exhibit increased uptake in response to stress.
- CT coronary angiography: improvements in the spatial resolution of CT scanning have allowed it to be used in the assessment of coronary artery disease. It can detect stenosis in the coronary arteries and also the degree of calcification within the walls of the vessels, which has been shown to correlate with the degree of stenosis.

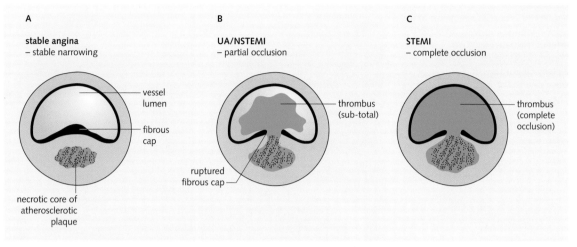

Fig. 7.6 The changes in the atherosclerotic plaque and associated thrombus underlying each of the manifestations of coronary artery disease. (A) Stable angina: atherosclerotic plaque with solid fibrous cap reducing the vessel lumen size. (B) UA/NSTEMI: ruptured fibrous cap with partially occlusive thrombus formation. (C) STEMI: ruptured fibrous cap with complete vessel occlusion by thrombus (UA, unstable angina; NSTEMI, non-ST elevation myocardial infarction; STEMI, ST elevation myocardial infarction).

- Coronary angiography (Figs 7.7 and 7.8): visualization of the patency of the coronary vasculature using intravenous contrast to assess the location and extent of coronary artery stenosis. The procedure is performed by passing a catheter through the aorta via the femoral or radial artery to the origins of the coronary arteries and injecting a contrast agent.

Treatment

Pharmacological treatment of angina

Treatment strategies for angina aim to restore the balance between myocardial supply and demand by increasing blood supply, and therefore oxygen supply, to the ischaemic myocardium and decreasing the oxygen demand of the myocardium (Fig. 7.9).

Increasing blood supply can be achieved by:

- Decreasing heart rate: coronary artery flow occurs primarily during diastole. Decreasing heart rate prolongs diastole allowing more time for perfusion of the myocardium.
- Dilating coronary arteries: this may be of more benefit in angina due to coronary artery spasm as stenosed coronary arteries are likely to be already maximally vasodilated by endogenous metabolic vasodilators (such as adenosine).

Decreasing the oxygen demand of the myocardium can be achieved by:

- Decreasing heart rate.
- Decreasing contractility.
- Decreasing preload.
- Decreasing afterload.

Organic nitrates

Organic nitrates, e.g. glyceryl trinitrate (GTN), relax vascular smooth muscle by producing nitric oxide (NO), which increases levels of cGMP and brings about dilatation. Nitrates mediate their effects by:

- Dilatation of venous capacitance vessels (predominant effect): this causes pooling of blood in the venous system which:
  - Reduces the preload of the heart and according to Starling's law, decreased preload leads to decreased cardiac output, decreasing myocardial work.
  - Decreases arterial blood pressure, thus reducing the afterload.
- Dilatation of coronary arteries: nitrates have a direct vasodilatory effect on coronary arteries at high doses, increasing myocardial perfusion.

GTN is usually administered sublingually to avoid first pass metabolism and its effects last around 30 minutes. Tolerance develops to the effects of GTN if used regularly over 2 or 3 days and patients should be aware of this. It can be used to relieve an attack or can be taken prophylactically to prevent an attack. Longer acting nitrates include isosorbide mononitrate and isosorbide dinitrate. The side-effects of nitrates include postural hypotension and sometimes a reflex tachycardia as the body attempts to maintain blood pressure. Headaches and facial flushing can also occur.

Calcium channel blockers (e.g. nifedipine, verapamil, diltiazem)

These drugs block L-type Ca^{2+} channels and have effects on both the heart and arteriolar smooth muscle:

Fig. 7.7 Coronary angiograms of normal left (A) and right (B) coronary arteries, each taken in two perpendicular views. (Courtesy of Newby DE, Grubb NR. Cardiology: an illustrated colour text. Edinburgh: Elsevier, 2005.)

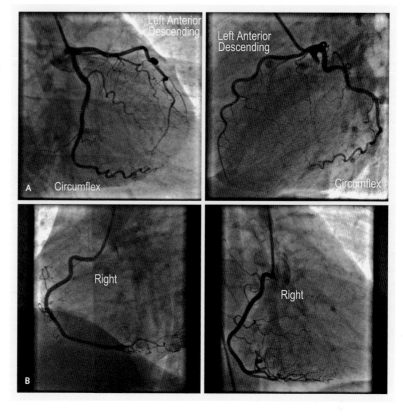

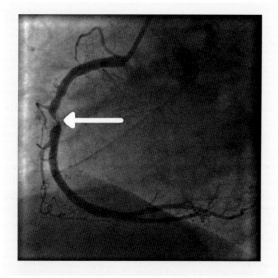

Fig. 7.8 Coronary angiogram of a patient with a severe coronary stenosis (arrow). (Courtesy of Newby D E, Grubb N R. Cardiology: an illustrated colour text. Edinburgh: Elsevier, 2005.)

- Blockade of myocardial L-type Ca^{2+} channels (greatest with non-dyhydropyridine agents, verapamil and diltiazem):
  - Decreases heart rate by decreasing the slope of the pacemaker potential and action potential upstroke in the sinoatrial node (SAN) and increasing delay at the atrioventricular node (AVN). Remember these drugs are also class IV antiarrhythmics.
  - Decreases the Ca^{2+} influx during the plateau of the ventricular action potential, therefore decreasing contractility and myocardial oxygen demand.
- Blockade of L-type Ca^{2+} channels in vascular smooth muscle (greatest with dihydropyridine agents such as nifedipine and amlodipine):
  - Direct dilatation of coronary arteries increases myocardial perfusion.
  - Peripheral vasodilatation decreases arterial blood pressure, decreasing afterload and myocardial work.

Owing to their negative chronotropic effects, care must be taken when using verapamil or diltiazem in combination with beta-blockers, as profound bradycardia may result. Nifedipine, however, may be beneficially combined with beta-blockers to minimize reflex tachycardia.

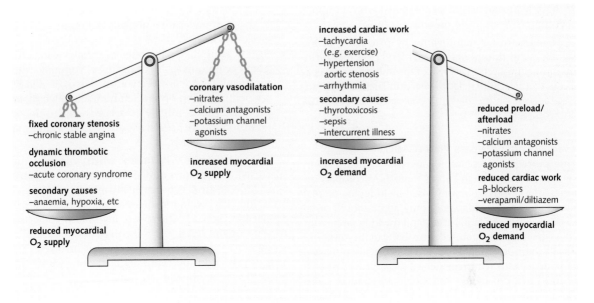

Fig. 7.9 Balance of myocardial oxygen supply and demand in ischaemic heart disease, and the rationale for the use of antianginal therapies. (Courtesy of Newby DE, Grubb NR. Cardiology: an illustrated colour text. Edinburgh: Elsevier, 2005.)

Beta-blockers (e.g. atenolol, metoprolol)

These drugs block sympathetic stimulation of the heart, leading to:

- Decreased contractility (negative inotropic effect) and, therefore, decreased oxygen demand.
- Decreased heart rate and, therefore, decreased oxygen demand and prolonged diastole, increasing duration of coronary blood flow.

They should be used with care in patients with asthma as blockade of bronchial β_2 receptors causes bronchoconstriction and may precipitate an attack. Care should be taken in patients with bradyarrhythmias and in patients with peripheral arterial disease, as they will reduce blood pressure and may impair perfusion of the peripheries.

> **HINTS AND TIPS**
>
> Many drugs of the same class have similar suffixes to their names. For example, most beta-blockers end in '-olol' (e.g. propranolol, atenolol, metoprolol). This is useful when identifying the class of an unfamiliar drug.

Nicorandil

Nicorandil is a potassium channel agonist that affects ATP-dependent K^+ channels in vascular smooth muscle, causing hyperpolarization and vasodilatation. It affects both arteries and veins, thus reducing both preload and afterload. Nicorandil also has a nitrate component, in that it is a nitric oxide donor. Nicorandil is not used first line but is an alternative to nitrates when tolerance occurs and if beta-blockers and Ca^{2+} antagonists are contraindicated.

Ivabradine

A new agent that inhibits the pacemaker potential in the SA node, slowing the rate of depolarization and reducing heart rate.

Interventional treatments

Percutaneous coronary intervention (PCI)

PCI describes a number of procedures to relieve stenosis in the coronary arteries performed by insertion of a catheter, usually via the femoral artery. Percutaneous treatment options for coronary artery disease include:

- Balloon angioplasty: an inflatable balloon is passed into the affected coronary artery and inflated within the stenosis, compressing it and expanding the lumen.
- Metal stents: a metallic stent is positioned within the stenosis, expanding the vessel walls and restoring vessel patency. Stents decrease the need for reintervention when compared with balloon angioplasty but the stents put pressure on the wall of the artery causing endothelial damage and stimulating a proliferative response. This proliferative response causes scar tissue deposition that can cause narrowing of the expanded lumen. Attempts to overcome this

have led to the use of stents coated with immuno-suppressive agents to prevent re-stenosis.

Damage to the endothelium by placement of the stent is highly thrombogenic and blood clots may form, occluding the artery. This risk of thrombosis means patients require antiplatelet medication such as clopido-grel, aspirin or the newer agents such as GPIIb/IIIa antagonists (see p. 99).

Coronary artery bypass graft (CABG)

This procedure uses autologous (the patient's own) veins and/or arteries to bypass stenosis in coronary arteries. The vessels commonly used include the internal mammary artery, which is directly anastamosed distal to the stenosis, the radial artery and the long saphenous vein which are anastamosed proximally to the aorta and distally beyond the stenosis. CABG is usually indicated in patients with left main stem disease or triple-vessel disease, while patients with single- or double-vessel disease are usually treated with PCI. The procedure is traditionally performed with the patients on a cardio-pulmonary bypass machine. In recent years, however, some surgeons have been performing this procedure without putting patients on bypass (so called 'off pump' CABG). Generally, although CABG is associated with higher short-term mortality and morbidity, the need for subsequent reintervention is less than with PCI.

Acute coronary syndromes

Angina is in effect the chronic manifestation of coronary artery disease and results from stable atherosclerotic plaques that cause stenosis of coronary arteries. The acute manifestations of coronary artery disease are termed acute coronary syndromes and occur when the fibrous cap of an atherosclerotic plaque becomes unstable and one of the following occurs (Fig. 7.6):

- Plaque erosion: this occurs when there is damage to the endothelium overlying the plaque. This exposes the prothrombotic subendothelial connective tissue, causing platelet adhesion and formation of a throm-bus on the surface of the plaque, which can occlude the lumen. The sequence of events in thrombus for-mation is shown in Fig. 7.10.
- Plaque rupture/fissure: this occurs in advanced pla-que when deep fissures form in the plaque allowing blood to flow into the plaque. A thrombus then forms within the plaque causing it to expand and occlude the vessel lumen.

Clinically, these acute plaque changes can manifest as one of three acute coronary syndromes, in order of increasing severity:

- Unstable angina (UA): angina of increasing severity or at rest without evidence of myocardial necrosis.

- NSTEMI: new onset chest pain with biochemical evidence of myocardial necrosis but no ST segment elevation on ECG.
- STEMI: acute chest pain, often associated with auto-nomic symptoms such as sweating or vomiting, with biochemical evidence of myocardial necrosis and ST segment elevation or new left bundle branch block on ECG. This is usually associated with complete occlusion of the coronary artery and significant myocardial necrosis.

Myocardial infarction occurs when myocytes die (necrosis) due to myocardial ischaemia. Irreversible damage occurs from between 20–40 minutes after vessel occlusion. The evolution of infarcted myocardium is depicted in Fig. 7.11. The area of myocardium affected depends on the vessel that is involved and the changes on the ECG allow assessment of the area involved. The area of infarction following occlusion of each of the major vessels is shown in Fig. 7.12.

Biochemical markers of myocyte necrosis

Myocyte necrosis can be detected biochemically by mea-suring levels of cardiac enzymes (creatine kinase and lactate dehydrogenase) and cardiac troponin T and I. A rise in these markers suggests myocardial necrosis and therefore infarction. In NSTEMI, there can be an increase in these markers but they are usually significantly elevated in STEMI. The timing and duration of the rise of each of these markers after myocardial infarction is depicted in Fig. 7.13.

> Myocardial necrosis is not the only cause of a raised troponin. Troponin can be raised owing to:
> - Pulmonary embolism.
> - Sepsis.
> - Renal failure.
> - Arrhythmia.

Investigations

- ECG: in UA/NSTEMI, ST segment depression and T wave inversion (similar to during an attack of an-gina) may be present. Be aware that in these, the ECG may be completely normal. In STEMI, ST eleva-tion or new left bundle branch block must be present to make the diagnosis. Fig. 7.14 shows ST segment elevation and the subsequent changes seen on ECG in the days/weeks following a STEMI.
- Cardiac enzymes.

Management

Immediate management of all patients with ACS should be administration of analgesia (usually morphine), aspirin, clopidogrel and a beta-blocker (explained

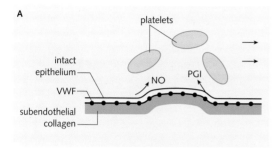

The continuous endothelial layer prevents circulating platelets from coming into contact with the prothrombotic subendothelial components
- von-Willebrand factor (VWF)
- Collagen

The intact endothelium prevents activation of platelets by secretion of nitric oxide and prostacyclin.

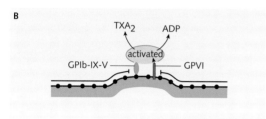

Subendothelial von-Willebrand factor tether platelets on platelet surface receptor GPIb – IX – V. Firm adhesion to subendothelial collagen via GPVI activates the platelet and stimulates release of ADP and synthesis of Thromboxane A_2 (TXA_2).

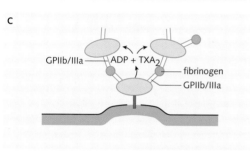

Binding of GPVI also induces expression and activation of platelet integrin GPIIb/IIIa, which binds to fibrinogen. The ADP and TXA_2 released activates other platelets, inducing expression of GPIIb/IIIa, and allowing platelet cross linking via fibrinogen. Activation of platelets causes further release of ADP and TXA_2 causing a positive feedback effect.

The aggregation of platelets provides a prothrombotic surface for the clotting/coagulation cascade. The coagulation cascade (D) results in formation of fibrin which forms a mesh around and between the aggregated platelets. This end result is a clot.

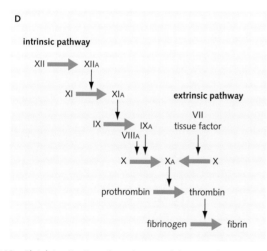

Fig. 7.10 Platelet activation, thrombosis and the coagulation cascade (VWF, von-Willebrand factor; ADP, adenosine diphosphate; TXA_2, thromboxane A_2; GP, glycoprotein; NO, nitric oxide; PGI, prostacyclin).

below). If they are hypoxic they should be given oxygen, but oxygen is not currently recommended for all patients routinely. The subsequent management is dependent on the presence of ST elevation and is shown in the algorithm in Fig. 7.15.

Drugs used in the treatment of ACS

Antiplatelet agents

Antiplatelet agents aim to prevent further activation and aggregation of platelets, reducing the likelihood of expansion of the thrombus occluding the affected coronary artery. A number of agents are available.

Fig. 7.11 Morphological changes occurring following myocardial infarction

time	macroscopic appearance	microscopic appearance
0–12 hours	not visible	infarcted muscle appears uncoloured on staining with nitroblue tetrazolium due to loss of oxidative enzymes; non-infarcted muscle stains blue
12-24 hours	pale with blotchy discolouration	infarcted muscle is brightly eosinophilic with intercellular oedema
24–72 hours	dead area appears soft and pale with a slight yellow colour	infarcted area excites an acute inflammatory response neutrophils infiltrate between dead cardiac muscle fibres
3–10 days	hyperaemic border develops around the yellow dead muscle	organization of infarcted area replacement with vascular granulation tissue
weeks to months	white scar	progressive collagen deposition infarct is replaced by a collagenous scar

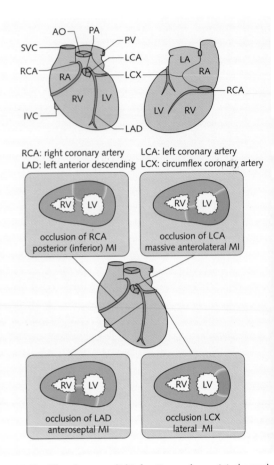

RCA: right coronary artery LCA: left coronary artery
LAD: left anterior descending LCX: circumflex coronary artery

Fig. 7.12 Site of myocardial infarction and associated vessel involvement.

When thinking about antiplatelet agents, consider at which stage of the platelet thrombus formation they act. Both aspirin and clopidogrel are given to patients with ACS because they inhibit the process of platelet aggregation at two points, and thus have a greater effect than one of the drugs alone.

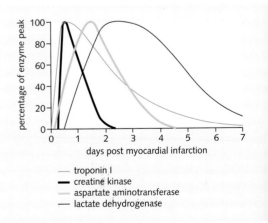

Fig. 7.13 Schematic profile of the release of cardiac enzyme and markers. (Courtesy of Newby DE, Grubb NR. Cardiology an illustrated colour text. Edinburgh: Elsevier, 2005.)

Aspirin

Aspirin is the most important antiplatelet drug in the treatment of coronary artery disease. It irreversibly inhibits the enzyme cyclooxygenase (COX) which is involved in the synthesis of the potent platelet activator thromboxane A_2 (TXA_2) from arachidonic acid. COX is also involved in the synthesis of prostacyclin (PGI_2), which exerts inhibitory effects on platelet function. PGI_2 synthesis is also blocked by aspirin, but the endothelial cells, which produce mainly PGI_2, are able to produce more COX enzyme (this cannot occur in platelets as they have no nucleus), leading to the balance shifting towards production of the antiplatelet PGI_2. Side-effects of aspirin include an increased risk of bleeding due to inhibited platelet function and it can cause gastric irritation leading to stomach ulcers. Aspirin can also be used in primary and secondary prevention of coronary artery disease by preventing thrombosis.

> **HINTS AND TIPS**
>
> Primary prevention describes measures aimed at preventing an unaffected person from developing a disease. Secondary prevention describes measures aimed at preventing progression and future events in a person who is already suffering from a disease.

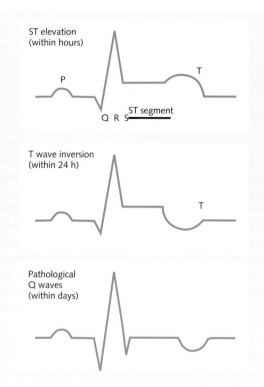

Fig. 7.14 ECG trace showing a STEMI with ST segment elevation and the subsequent evolution of ECG changes that follow a STEMI.

Clopidogrel

Clopidogrel is a thienopyridine derivative and is given to all patients with ACS. The mechanism of action of clopidogrel is irreversible blockade of the adenosine diphosphate (ADP) receptor on platelet cell membranes. This receptor is named P2Y12 and is important in platelet aggregation. The blockade of this receptor inhibits platelet aggregation by blocking activation of the glycoprotein IIb/IIIa pathway. New agents such as ticagrelor inhibit the same receptor but do so reversibly.

GPIIb/IIIa inhibitors

These agents inhibit the binding of fibrinogen to GPIIb/IIIa receptors on activated platelets, thus inhibiting platelet aggregation. Examples include eptifibatide and abciximab. These drugs are only used in ACS for high-risk patients and those undergoing urgent PCI.

Anticoagulant agents

All patients with UA or NSTEMI should receive low molecular weight heparin by subcutaneous injection. This inhibits the coagulation cascade by inhibiting factor Xa.

Beta-blockers

Administration of beta-blockers decreases heart rate and myocardial work. They have been repeatedly demonstrated to be beneficial in patients following ACS and should be continued long term.

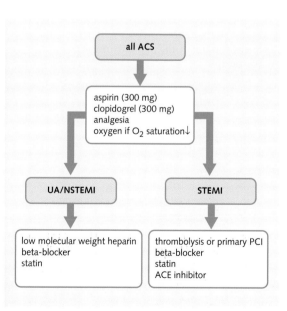

Fig. 7.15 Algorithm for the treatment of acute coronary syndromes.

Thrombolytic therapy

Thrombolytic (fibrinolytic) therapy is used to break down the thrombi that cause myocardial infarction and allow reperfusion of the affected area. These agents achieve this by converting plasmin to the fibrinolytic enzyme plasminogen, which breaks down the fibrin mesh that binds a thrombus together. They are only used in STEMI when primary PCI is not available and must be administered by a senior doctor after careful assessment for the presence of contraindications. The administration of thrombolytic agents should be followed by an infusion of heparin for 48 h to prevent recurrent thrombus formation and ischaemic events.

Thrombolytic agents include:

- Tissue plasminogen activators (TPA), e.g. tenecteplase, reteplase: these are the primary agents of choice for thrombolysis.
- Streptokinase: rarely used in clinical practice now. It binds and activates plasminogen to form plasmin, causing fibrinolysis. Plasmin also lyses fibrinogen and prothrombin (anticoagulant effect). Streptokinase cannot be used repeatedly as antibodies are generated which may induce anaphylaxis on subsequent exposure.

Indications for thrombolysis:
- Typical history of ischaemic cardiac chest pain less than 12 h duration
  AND
- 1 mm ST segment elevation in at least two adjacent limb leads on ECG, OR
- 2 mm ST segment elevation in at least two adjacent chest leads on ECG, OR
- New onset left bundle branch block.

Important contraindications to thrombolysis:
- Trauma with risk of haemorrhage.
- Recent surgery.
- Suspected aortic dissection.
- Pregnancy.
- Recent stroke (within 6 months).
- Active bleeding.

Primary PCI

Most centres now use angioplasty or stenting to relieve the blockage and allow reperfusion of the myocardium. Primary PCI describes the situation when PCI is the initial definitive treatment and thrombolytic agents have not been administered. When thrombolysis has been unsuccessful and PCI is performed this is called rescue PCI. When the facilities to perform primary PCI are available, it is preferred to thrombolysis because of the risk of significant bleeding with thrombolysis.

Complications

Sudden death (within 6 h of symptom onset) occurs in 25% of patients following STEMI, usually as a result of arrhythmia. In those who survive this initial period, MI can lead to a number of acute and chronic complications. The major ones include:

- Heart failure: infarcted myocardium is unable to contract effectively.
- Arrhythmia.
- Myocardial rupture: this can be either the free wall of a ventricle or the interventricular septum and can be rapidly fatal without emergency surgical intervention.
- Mitral regurgitation: owing to infarction and subsequent rupture of the papillary muscles.
- Pericarditis.

Heart failure, myocardial and pericardial disease (8)

Objectives

You should be able to:
- Understand the definition of heart failure and its different forms.
- Describe the causes of heart failure.
- Understand the compensatory responses to impaired ventricular function.
- Understand how these changes become maladaptive and give rise to the syndrome of heart failure.
- Understand the origin and character of the most common arrhythmias.
- Describe the clinical features of heart failure.
- Describe the drugs used in the treatment of heart failure and the rationale for their use.
- Understand the three forms of cardiomyopathy.
- Describe the common diseases involving the pericardium.
- Understand the causes of cardiac tamponade and the associated clinical signs.

HEART FAILURE

Heart failure (cardiac failure) is the clinical syndrome that arises when the heart is no longer able to maintain sufficient tissue perfusion to meet the metabolic demands of the body's tissues, despite normal filling pressures. Heart failure is a serious condition that carries a very poor prognosis: 20–30% of patients will die within 1 year and 60% will be dead within 5 years. This is a worse prognosis than many cancers.

In most patients with heart failure, it occurs as a result of decreased stroke volume due to impaired systolic function (contractility) of the left ventricle. The ejection fraction is usually reduced (<50%) and it may be referred to as low output heart failure or heart failure with reduced ejection fraction. In this situation, the reduction in contractility means the Starling curve is shifted downwards (Fig. 8.1) such that stroke volume is reduced for any given end-diastolic pressure (EDP).

Low output heart failure can also be caused by diastolic dysfunction in situations where ventricular filling is impaired. This limits the end-diastolic volume (EDV) and thus stroke volume and cardiac output. In diastolic dysfunction, ventricular compliance is usually decreased and the relationship between EDV and EDP becomes non-linear. As a result, the Starling curve is no longer valid. The relationship between EDV and stroke volume, however, is still valid. In this situation, EDV is restricted, restricting stroke volume, but the ejection fraction is preserved. This is sometimes referred to as heart failure with preserved ejection fraction.

The final situation that can bring about heart failure is when the metabolic demands of the body are persistently increased and the heart is unable to maintain sufficient cardiac output. This is called high output heart failure and can occur in severe anaemia, thyrotoxicosis and sepsis. It is unusual if the heart is structurally and functionally normal but can precipitate heart failure in a structurally abnormal or diseased heart.

Causes of heart failure

Conditions that lead to heart failure can be broadly divided into:

1. Those that damage cardiac muscle itself

- Ischaemic heart disease: this is somewhat of a misnomer because it is actually infarction that is more likely to cause heart failure. An infarcted segment

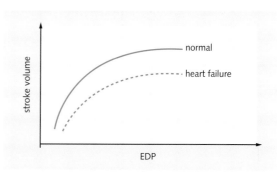

Fig. 8.1 The Starling curve in heart failure. Reduced contractility reduces stroke volume for a given filling pressure (EDP, end-diastolic pressure).

of ventricle is unable to contract effectively, decreasing systolic function.

- Cardiomyopathy: whether it causes impaired systolic or diastolic dysfunction, cardiomyopathy can cause heart failure. Cardiomyopathy is discussed further below.
- Myocarditis: depending on the cause and clinical course, myocarditis can cause acute heart failure or heart failure some time after the myocarditis has resolved.

2. Those that demand extra work of the heart

- Hypertension: chronically increased afterload leads to compensatory left ventricular hypertrophy. This impairs diastolic filling due to decreased ventricular compliance and increases the myocardial oxygen demand.
- Valvular heart disease: can cause either pressure overload (e.g. aortic stenosis) or volume overload (e.g. aortic regurgitation or mitral regurgitation) in the left ventricle decreasing efficiency.
- Severe anaemia, thyrotoxicosis and arteriovenous fistulas all place extra demands on the heart.

These processes most commonly affect the left ventricle, but isolated right ventricular failure can occur in some circumstances. Remember that the most common cause of right ventricular failure is left ventricular failure. Causes of isolated right ventricular failure include:

- Right ventricular myocardial infarction.
- Cor pulmonale: this is right ventricular failure due to disease of the pulmonary vasculature. It can be

caused by recurrent pulmonary emboli, primary pulmonary hypertension or any respiratory disease in which there is persistent widespread hypoxic pulmonary vasoconstriction such as chronic obstructive pulmonary disease (COPD). All of these conditions increase pulmonary vascular resistance causing pressure and volume overload of the right ventricle.

Decreased right ventricular cardiac output limits left ventricular preload and thus left ventricular stroke volume which can bring about the same responses as those that occur when the left ventricle is primarily affected.

HINTS AND TIPS

Remember, 'heart failure' is NOT a diagnosis. It is always necessary to identify the underlying pathology responsible, so that a targeted treatment regimen can be employed.

Compensatory mechanisms

When stroke volume and cardiac output are reduced due to either systolic or diastolic dysfunction there are a number of compensatory changes (Fig. 8.2) that occur to restore cardiac output and maintain tissue perfusion. These changes are successful initially (adaptive). The decrease in stroke volume reduces arterial blood pressure causing unloading of the arterial baroreceptors. This brings about a number of changes including:

- Increased sympathetic and decreased parasympathetic outflow to the heart increasing heart rate

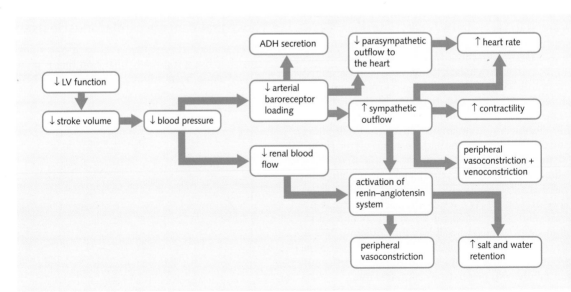

Fig. 8.2 Compensatory adaptations to impaired left ventricular function (LV, left ventricular; ADH, antidiuretic hormone).

and increasing contractility (the degree to which this can occur may be limited in a diseased myocardium).

- Increased sympathetic outflow to the peripheral vasculature causing vasoconstriction to increase total peripheral resistance and venoconstriction, limiting venous pooling and increasing venous return.
- Antidiuretic hormone (ADH) secretion is increased from the posterior pituitary increasing water reabsorption in the renal collecting ducts.
- Decreased renal blood flow and increased sympathetic outflow to the kidneys increases release of renin. This increases angiotensin II (and thus aldosterone) levels causing further peripheral vasoconstriction and promoting salt and water retention in the kidneys.

These changes increase circulating volume and cardiac filling pressures, which increases stroke volume by virtue of Starling's law and increases heart rate and total peripheral resistance (TPR), which together maintain arterial blood pressure and tissue perfusion. In the early stages, these changes are able to compensate for the impaired cardiac function and clinical manifestations of heart failure may be minimal.

The vicious cycle of heart failure

As systolic dysfunction progresses and these compensatory mechanisms persist and intensify they become maladaptive, accelerate disease progression and bring about the clinical syndrome of heart failure (Fig. 8.3):

- Persistent activation of the renin–angiotensin system and ADH release causes further fluid retention. Initially in place to increase filling pressures to maximize stroke volume, filling pressures become excessive and stroke volume decreases due to overstretching of the myocytes. This moves the heart onto the downward part of the Starling curve.
- The increased filling pressures and ventricular pressures will cause congestion in the pulmonary circulation causing alveolar oedema (due to left ventricular (LV) backpressure) and in the systemic veins causing peripheral oedema (due to right ventricular (RV) backpressure).
- These excessive filling pressures cause dilatation of the ventricular walls. As the ventricles distend, the afterload increases according to Laplace's law. As this dilatation progresses, it can also cause disruption of the atrioventricular (mitral and tricuspid) valve annulus and cause valvular regurgitation.
- The persistent tachycardia reduces the duration of diastole and thus the duration of coronary blood flow. With the increase in contractility, myocardial oxygen demand is increased while oxygen delivery is reduced. These two factors combined may cause myocardial ischaemia, which will further impair function.
- Persistently high levels of angiotensin II, aldosterone and catecholamines bring about a process of left ventricular remodelling causing changes in cardiac metabolism, myocardial thinning and fibrosis.

Clinical features

Many of the symptoms and signs of heart failure are due to reduced cardiac output, volume overload and increased pressures within the circulation. Left ventricular failure will result in increased congestion into the pulmonary circulation, and can cause further backpressure

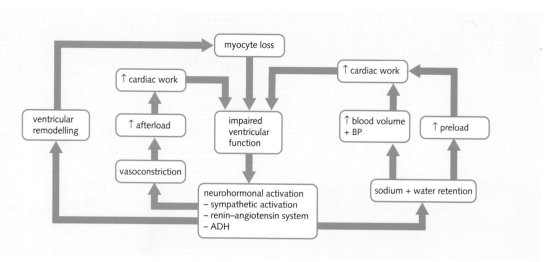

Fig. 8.3 The vicious cycle of heart failure (BP, blood pressure; ADH, antidiuretic hormone).

Fig. 8.4 The clinical signs of heart failure. Separated into general signs and those caused by left ventricular and right ventricular failure.

Left-sided	Right-sided	General
• Bibasal pulmonary crackles	• Elevated JVP	• Pale peripheries
• Pleural effusions	• Ankle oedema	• Tachycardia
• Murmur of mitral regurgitation	• Sacral oedema	• Low volume pulse
	• Hepatomegaly	• Cachexia
	• Murmur of tricuspid regurgitation	

and congestion into the systemic venous circulation. Right ventricular failure on the other hand, does not cause pulmonary congestion, but does cause congestion of the systemic veins. Fig. 8.4 depicts the clinical signs of heart failure.

Symptoms include:

- Fatigue.
- Dyspnoea: owing to alveolar oedema caused by pulmonary venous congestion.
- Orthopnoea: this is shortness of breath in the supine position. When supine, blood redistributes to the intrathoracic compartment increasing pressures and alveolar oedema. It can be relieved by sitting upright, and patients will often report that they have to sleep with multiple pillows.
- Paroxysmal nocturnal dyspnoea: patients wake up in the night gasping for breath.
- Swollen ankles: due to oedema from increased fluid filtration caused by increased venous pressure.
- Nocturia (urination during the night): as peripheral oedema is reabsorbed into the circulation when supine at night, circulating volume increases and is compensated for by an increase in urine output.

The severity of the symptoms and functional capacity of patients in heart failure are often described using the New York Heart Association classification (Fig. 8.5).

Signs include:

- Pale, cold peripheries: due to the persistent cutaneous vasoconstriction.

Fig. 8.5 NYHA functional classification for heart failure

Class I (mild)	No limitation of physical activity by symptoms
Class II (mild)	Symptoms with ordinary activity
Class III (moderate)	Symptoms with minimal activity
Class IV (severe)	Symptoms at rest

- Tachycardia: may be sinus tachycardia or 'irregularly irregular' pulse if in atrial fibrillation (AF).
- Raised jugular venous pressure: due to increased right atrial pressure from the overloaded right ventricle.
- Displaced apex impulse on palpation: if the left ventricle is dilated, the apex beat may be displaced inferiorly and laterally.
- A third and/or fourth heart sound may be present.
- Bi-basal pulmonary crackles: due to alveolar oedema.
- Bilateral pitting oedema.
- Hepatomegaly can develop owing to hepatic venous congestion.
- May be a pansystolic murmur of mitral or tricuspid regurgitation.
- Pleural effusions: these are often bilateral but if unilateral, they tend to occur on the right.

In addition to the signs and symptoms described above: patients with heart failure are prone to developing arrhythmias. Atrial fibrillation is common in heart failure and the abnormal ventricular myocardium predisposes to ventricular arrhythmias, which is the cause of death in a large proportion of these patients. Reduced blood pressure combined with renal vasoconstriction and use of angiotensin-converting enzyme (ACE) inhibitors puts these patients at an increased risk of developing pre-renal acute renal failure due to hypoperfusion.

Investigation may reveal the following:

- Electrocardiogram (ECG): may demonstrate atrial fibrillation, ventricular hypertrophy or left bundle branch block (LBBB). If the aetiology of the heart failure is ischaemic, there may be Q waves indicating a previous myocardial infarction with ST elevation (STEMI).
- Chest X-ray: may show an enlarged heart shadow due to dilatation and alveolar shadowing due to oedema. There may be small bilateral pleural effusions. A typical chest X-ray of a patient with chronic heart failure is shown in Fig. 8.6.
- Echocardiography: this is a key investigation in the assessment of heart failure. It allows quantification of the ejection fraction giving an indication of the degree of systolic dysfunction. Diastolic dysfunction can also be assessed. It also allows assessment of ventricular dilatation and valvular disease.
- B natriuretic peptide: this is released in response to ventricular stretch and is a very sensitive marker for heart failure.

Treatment of heart failure

The aims when treating heart failure include the following:

- Decrease preload.
- Decrease afterload by reducing both ventricular volume and blood pressure.

limits the degree of ventricular remodelling, reduces the afterload on the heart (by removing its vasoconstrictor effect) and limits salt and water retention. ACE inhibitors have been repeatedly demonstrated to improve survival and symptoms in heart failure and should be prescribed to everyone with heart failure whether symptomatic or not. If ACE inhibitors are not tolerated owing to dry cough, angiotensin II receptor antagonists can be used with equal efficacy.

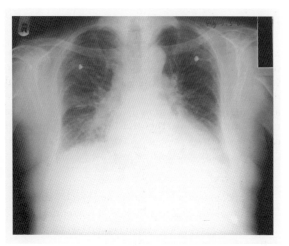

Fig. 8.6   Radiograph of the chest showing early pulmonary congestion. Note that the width of the heart shadow is greater than half the transthoracic diameter and that there are distended hila with increased lung markings. This indicates heart failure and pulmonary congestion. (Courtesy of Newby DE, Grubb NR. Cardiology: an illustrated colour text. Edinburgh: Elsevier, 2005.)

- Reverse or limit ventricular remodelling.
- Limit heart rate.

General measures

Patients with heart failure should restrict their intake of salt and if they are volume overloaded fluid restriction may also be useful. Alcohol should be avoided due to its toxic effects on the heart. Patients should also have their co-morbidities effectively managed.

Diuretics

Diuretics increase salt and water excretion in the kidneys. Loop diuretics such as furosemide are the class most widely used in heart failure to reduce circulating volume (and thus preload), reducing pulmonary congestion and peripheral oedema. Thiazide-like diuretics may also be added if loop diuretics alone are not effective in relieving symptoms. Unlike many of the other drugs used in heart failure, diuretics do not improve survival; they do, however, provide effective symptomatic relief. The exception to this statement is aldosterone antagonists, which have diuretic function but do improve prognosis, and are discussed below.

Angiotensin-converting enzyme inhibitors

ACE inhibitors (e.g. enalapril, lisinopril and captopril) inhibit production of angiotensin II (AgII) by angiotensin-converting enzyme. Inhibition of AgII in heart failure

Beta-blockers

The benefits of beta-blockers in heart failure include reduction in heart rate, increasing coronary blood flow. They also decrease the metabolic demand of the myocardium. In combination with ACE inhibitors, beta-blockers improve survival and reverse ventricular remodelling. In some cases, the decreased contractility and heart rate may worsen symptoms, so they should be introduced at low doses and the dose increased slowly.

Aldosterone antagonists

Aldosterone antagonists such as spironolactone and eplerenone have been shown to improve survival in heart failure. They reduce preload by inhibiting the action of aldosterone in the renal tubules. They do, however, increase the risk of life-threatening hyperkalaemia, especially when used in combination with an ACE inhibitor, so electrolyte levels must be closely monitored. Spironolactone may also cause painful gynaecomastia.

Cardiac glycosides

Digoxin is an inhibitor of the $Na^+/K^+ATPase$. This causes accumulation of Ca^{2+} in the cytosol of the myocytes exerting a positive inotropic effect. It also acts centrally, increasing vagal outflow to the heart, decreasing heart rate. The use of digoxin is recommended in patients with heart failure if they have atrial fibrillation to control the heart rate and in patients with severe heart failure.

Nitrates

Glyceryl trinitrate (GTN) relaxes vascular smooth muscle by increasing levels of cGMP. It preferentially dilates venous vessels and its use in heart failure is usually limited to the acute setting because tolerance to its effects develops over 1 or 2 days. By dilating the venous vessels, GTN decreases preload, reducing the degree of ventricular volume overload.

Inotropic drugs

Inotropic drugs increase the contractility of the myocardium. Their principal role should be restricted to the management of acute heart failure, as they are associated with increased mortality with long-term use.

β₁-Sympathomimetics

The β1-sympathomimetics dobutamine and dopamine increase the force of myocardial contraction and heart rate. They are also vasodilators, reducing afterload.

Phosphodiesterase inhibitors

Milrinone inhibits phosphodiesterase type III, which is the enzyme that breaks down cyclic adenosine monophosphate (cAMP) into $5'$-AMP. Inhibition causes a rise in intracellular cAMP and, therefore, Ca^{2+}. This means there is an increase in contractility. Milrinone is also a vasodilator by the same mechanism in vascular smooth muscle. It is used in severe heart failure that is unresponsive to other therapy.

Device therapy

Cardiac resynchronization therapy (CRT)

Patients with heart failure often have left bundle branch block. As the conduction system in these individuals is abnormal, the ventricles do not contract uniformly (there is some dyssynchrony in the ventricular contraction). New pacemakers have been developed that stimulate both the right and the left ventricle simultaneously, with the obvious benefit of resynchronizing the left and right ventricles. This increases cardiac output and is of benefit in patients with heart failure and broad QRS complexes.

Implantable cardiac defibrillators (ICDs)

Patients with heart failure are prone to life-threatening arrhythmias (e.g. ventricular tachycardia (VT), ventricular fibrillation (VF)). ICDs can be implanted in a similar way to pacemaker devices to deliver a small electrical impulse when an arrhythmia arises, preventing sudden cardiac death. These devices can also prevent tachyarrhythmias by override pacing.

Ventricular assist device

Implantation of mechanical ventricular assist devices which take over the work of the failing ventricle can be used as a temporary solution until transplantation can be performed or until the ventricle recovers its function.

Transplantation

Heart transplantation is the only definitive treatment for severe, intractable heart failure. The procedure requires life-long immunosuppression, which puts patients at increased risk of infection. With good patient selection, the prognosis is good, with 1-year survival rates of 80% and 5-year survival of 70%. The quality of life of the majority of patients is dramatically improved.

DISEASES OF THE MYOCARDIUM

Myocardial damage can be caused by a number of pathological processes. Ischaemia/infarction, arrhythmia, valvular disease and hypertension all cause myocardial damage and have been discussed elsewhere. There are also a number of conditions that cause intrinsic damage to the myocardium. These include myocarditis and cardiomyopathy.

> **HINTS AND TIPS**
>
> Cardiomyopathy and myocarditis are, in comparison to ischaemic heart disease, very rare. It is important to bear this in mind when learning about conditions that affect the cardiovascular system.

Myocarditis

Myocarditis is inflammation of the myocardium. Causes include:

- Infection: viruses (coxsackie, influenza, rubella, echovirus, polio); bacteria (*Corynebacterium* – diphtheria, *Rickettsia*, *Chlamydia*); protozoa (*Trypanosoma cruzi* – Chagas' disease, *Toxoplasma gondii*); fungi (*Candida*).
- Immune-mediated reactions: after infections (viral or rheumatic fever); systemic lupus erythematosus; transplant rejection; chemicals, radiation and drugs (chloroquine, methyldopa, lead poisoning).

Cardiomyopathy

Cardiomyopathy is often divided into the following three categories based on the morphological features of the diseased myocardium (Fig. 8.7):

- Dilated cardiomyopathy (85%): with dilated ventricles and impaired systolic function.
- Hypertrophic cardiomyopathy (10%): hypertrophy of ventricular myocardium, particularly the interventricular septum.
- Restrictive cardiomyopathy (5%): decreased ventricular compliance restricts ventricular filling.

Dilated cardiomyopathy

In contrast to the normal heart, dilated cardiomyopathy (DCM) causes dilated ventricles and poor systolic (contractile) function. Its prevalence is 0.2%. Causes of DCM include:

- Idiopathic: 30% have a familial element.
- Alcohol toxicity.

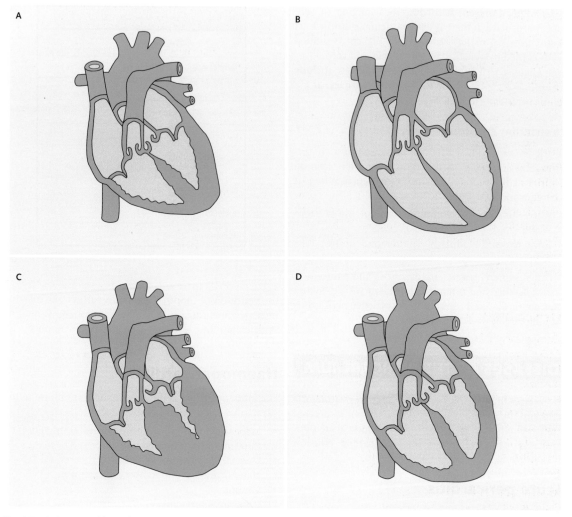

Fig. 8.7 (A) A normal heart for comparison with the cardiomyopathic hearts shown in B, C and D. (B) Dilated cardiomyopathy. The ventricles are thin and dilated. (C) Hypertrophic cardiomyopathy. There is an increase in ventricular mass. (D) Restrictive cardiomyopathy. The heart is of normal size, but the ventricles are stiff.

- Viral myocarditis: myocarditis can progress to dilated cardiomyopathy. The initial acute myocarditis may not have been noticed at the time.
- Peripartum: physiological changes during the final trimester of pregnancy can trigger the development of a DCM.
- Drugs: chemotherapeutic drugs (e.g. doxorubicin, trastuzumab).

The morphology of the heart in DCM is as follows:

- Thin, dilated walls in all chambers.
- Irregular myocyte hypertrophy and fibrosis.

Dilated ventricles may cause disruption of the atrioventricular valves causing regurgitation. DCM leads to heart failure, predisposes to arrhythmia, and patients often develop a mural thrombus in the left ventricle predisposing to embolic events.

Hypertrophic cardiomyopathy

Hypertrophic cardiomyopathy (HCM) is characterized by hypertrophy of the ventricles. The pattern of hypertrophy is variable but tends to preferentially affect the interventricular septum. In patients with septal hypertrophy adjacent to the left ventricular outflow tract, it can cause outflow tract obstruction. In these patients the condition is called hypertrophic obstructive cardiomyopathy (HOCM) and accounts for one third of cases of HCM. The disease leads to myocyte hypertrophy and disarray, disrupting ventricular contraction, and can cause abnormal mitral valve movement and mitral regurgitation. The hypertrophy reduces ventricular compliance impairing ventricular filling and causing diastolic dysfunction. About 50% of cases are inherited (autosomal dominant pattern) and the condition tends to manifest in early adulthood.

HCM may present with dyspnoea, angina or syncope, particularly if there is left ventricular outflow tract obstruction, but in many cases it may present as sudden death caused by ventricular arrhythmia and cardiac arrest. Characteristic findings on examination include a fourth heart sound (due to the stiff ventricle), and a systolic murmur (in HOCM).

Restrictive cardiomyopathy

Restrictive cardiomyopathy is a rare condition characterized by stiffening of the ventricular myocardium. The reduced compliance restricts ventricular filling. It is often associated with:

- Amyloidosis: most common form in the Western world.
- Endomyocardial fibrosis: children and young adults in Africa.

Patients often present with dyspnoea and reduced exercise tolerance and often develop heart failure. Symptoms are similar to those seen in constrictive pericarditis with impaired exercise tolerance.

DISEASES OF THE PERICARDIUM

The pericardium is the fibrous sac that surrounds the heart and the roots of the great vessels. Conditions that can arise involving the pericardium include acute pericarditis, constrictive pericarditis, pericardial effusion and cardiac tamponade.

Acute pericarditis

Pericarditis is an inflammation of the pericardium that leads to sharp retrosternal chest pain that radiates to the back, and that is aggravated by movement and respiration. On auscultation there may be a pericardial rub heard. Common causes are listed in Fig. 8.8. The mainstay of treatment is symptomatic relief with non-steroidal anti-inflammatory drugs. If the inflammatory process continues it can lead to fibrosis and shrinking of the pericardium (constrictive pericarditis) that can restrict cardiac filling. Constrictive pericarditis can also be caused by radiotherapy. The haemodynamic consequences of constrictive pericarditis are the same as those described below from cardiac tamponade but develop more slowly.

Pericardial effusion

A pericardial effusion is an accumulation of fluid in the pericardial cavity and can be caused by any condition causing pericarditis. The effusion collects in the closed cavity and causes distension. If the fluid accumulates slowly, the pericardium distends. If fluid accumulates quickly or

Fig. 8.8 Common causes of pericarditis
Viral (e.g. Coxsackie)
Tuberculosis
Trauma
Carcinoma (metastatic)
Uraemia
Myocardial infarction – acute – delayed (Dressler's)
Rheumatic fever
Bacterial
Rheumatoid arthritis

the pericardium cannot distend any further, the pressure increases and can cause cardiac tamponade (impaired ventricular filling leading to loss of cardiac output).

Haemopericardium

Haemopericardium is the accumulation of blood in the pericardial sac. It is caused by:

- Myocardial rupture after a myocardial infarction.
- Rupture of the intrapericardial aorta.
- Dissecting aortic aneurysm.
- Haemorrhage from an abscess or tumour.
- Trauma.

As with pericardial effusion, the consequences depend on the rate of accumulation of blood.

Cardiac tamponade

When fluid or blood accumulates quickly within the pericardial sac, the pericardium does not stretch and the increase in pressure effectively compresses the heart. The signs of cardiac tamponade are described by Beck's triad and include:

- Hypotension: increased pressure in the atria and ventricles impairs cardiac filling during diastole. This diastolic dysfunction limits the ventricular end-diastolic volume and thus stroke volume. This decreases cardiac output causing hypotension. If severe this can lead to shock.
- Raised jugular venous pressure (JVP): the increased pressure in the right atrium causes a raised JVP.
- Muffled/quiet heart sounds: the fluid around the heart reduces conduction of the heart sounds to the chest wall.

Another sign seen in cardiac tamponade is called Kussmaul's sign. This describes a paradoxical rise in the JVP during inspiration. During inspiration, the intrathoracic pressure decreases, effectively sucking blood into the intrathoracic compartment, increasing venous return. Usually this would increase right ventricular filling but in tamponade, this is prevented and causes a rise in the JVP.

Cardiac tamponade is a medical emergency and should be treated promptly by aspirating the blood/fluid from the pericardial space, a procedure called pericardiocentesis.

● Objectives

You should be able to:
- Understand the broad classification of arterial and venous disease.
- Describe the different manifestations of peripheral arterial disease.
- Understand the basic principles of examining the peripheral arterial system.
- Describe the main causes and types of aneurysms and the possible sequelae.
- Have a basic understanding of aortic dissection and carotid artery disease.
- Understand the two compartments of the lower limb venous system and the major pathology that affects each.
- Recall the risk factors for varicose veins and deep venous thrombosis.

ARTERIAL DISEASE

Arterial disease can be broadly divided into occlusive disease and aneurysmal disease.

Occlusive arterial disease

Chronic

This is commonly referred to as peripheral vascular disease and is caused by atherosclerosis in the major arteries supplying the lower limbs (rarely the upper limbs). As a result, the pathogenesis and risk factors for this disease are those that apply to atherosclerosis (see Ch. 7). People with coronary artery disease are likely to have a degree of peripheral vascular disease and vice versa because they are underpinned by the same pathological process.

Intermittent claudication

This is characterized by a 'gripping', cramp-like pain in the calf or buttock on exercise or walking, which subsides at rest. Stable angina is the coronary equivalent of intermittent claudication. It is due to an imbalance between oxygen supply and demand in the skeletal muscle. Atherosclerotic plaques in the arteries supplying the leg cause a stenosis, preventing the normal metabolically mediated increase in blood flow during exercise. As oxygen demand subsides with rest to a level such that blood flow is adequate once again, pain subsides. If pain is felt in the calf muscle, the blockage is usually in the femoral artery or the popliteal artery and if pain is felt in the buttocks, the blockage is usually more proximal, in the iliac artery.

At this relatively early stage in the disease, lifestyle modification to prevent disease progression is the mainstay of treatment. Patients should stop smoking, control blood pressure, diabetes and cholesterol pharmacologically, and try undertaking aerobic exercise as much as possible to promote development of collateral blood supply to the ischaemic muscle. If the symptoms are causing significant impact on the patient, angioplasty can be performed to dilate the stenosed vessel.

Critical limb ischaemia

This is characterized by pain at rest, gangrene, or an ankle–brachial pressure index less than 0.3 (discussed below). Rest pain occurs when blood flow to the affected muscle is limited to such a degree that it cannot provide adequate perfusion to meet the resting metabolic requirements of the muscle. Rest pain usually first occurs during the night when lower limb perfusion is not aided by gravity and patients may find relief by hanging their leg out of the bed.

> **HINTS AND TIPS**
>
> The features of critical limb ischaemia include:
> - Tissue loss.
> - Rest pain for >2 weeks.
> - Ankle–brachial pressure index (ABPI) <0.3.

Critical limb ischaemia can be treated in some cases with angioplasty, but often patients require surgery. Bypass surgery is often performed, in which a conduit (either a synthetic tube or the patient's long saphenous vein) is used to bypass the stenosed segment of artery, restoring perfusion. If symptoms cannot be controlled by bypass surgery, or gangrene has lead to severe infection, amputation of the limb may become necessary.

Acute limb ischaemia

Acute ischaemia occurs when there is acute occlusion of an artery. This is analogous to an acute coronary syndrome. In this case, unless there has been a history of chronic occlusive disease, there is unlikely to be much collateral circulation and blood flow to the distal tissues may be completely halted. Acute limb ischaemia presents with the 'six Ps' (three symptoms and three signs):

- Pain: due to skeletal muscle ischaemia.
- Paraesthesia: caused by ischaemia of the sensory nerves.
- Paralysis.
- Pallor.
- Pulselessness.
- Perishing cold (to touch).

  Causes of acute ischaemia include:

- Embolism: could originate from a thrombus in the heart in someone with atrial fibrillation, vegetations in someone with infective endocarditis or from a thrombus within the sac of an aneurysm (see below).
- Thrombosis: thrombosis of a ruptured atherosclerotic plaque (the equivalent of acute coronary syndrome).
- Raynaud's syndrome: excessive vasoconstriction, often in response to cold, prevents tissue perfusion. Most commonly affects the fingers.
- Trauma.

Examination

As with any examination, begin with inspection, comparing the two legs. Look for:

- Pallor.
- Ulcers: arterial ulcers tend to be deep and occur at points of pressure such as the heel and toes. It is also crucial to look between all the toes!
- Mottling of the skin.
- Hair loss.
- Scars.

Next, palpate both legs from top to bottom with the back of the hands to assess for any differences in temperature between the legs, or cold skin. Assess the capillary refill time in each foot by pressing firmly on the skin for 5 s, releasing your finger and observing the time it takes for the skin to return to its original colour. Normally the capillary refill time is less than 2 s.

Palpate the abdominal aorta, then palpate and auscultate (for bruits) each of the peripheral pulses as described below.

Femoral pulse

The femoral pulse is located just below the mid-inguinal point (halfway between the anterior superior iliac spine (ASIS) and the pubic symphysis). It is a strong pulse and should be easy to palpate.

Popliteal pulse

The popliteal arteries can be found in the popliteal fossae behind the knee and are often difficult to palpate. The thumbs of both hands should be rested on either side of the patella and the fingertips should be placed deep into the popliteal fossa so that the popliteal artery is compressed against the posterior aspect of the tibia. The popliteals are best palpated with the knees flexed at about 120°.

Posterior tibial pulse

The posterior tibial pulse is palpated about 1 cm posterior and inferior to the medial malleolus of the tibia with the patient's foot relaxed.

Dorsalis pedis pulse

The dorsalis pedis pulse is palpated against the tarsal bones on the dorsum of the foot, just lateral to the tendon of extensor hallucis longus.

Buerger's test

This is the final part of the examination for peripheral arterial disease. Start with the patient lying on the bed. Slowly lift each leg off the bed and observe the angle at which the leg goes pale, i.e. stops being adequately perfused. In normal individuals, the leg will remain perfused (and thus pink) all the way to 90° of hip flexion, but in patients with peripheral vascular disease, the leg may go pale at an angle of as little as 15°. A Buerger's angle of less than 20° indicates severe ischaemia. Having identified the Buerger's angle, lower the leg over the side of the bed and observe the colour change. In a patient with severe peripheral arterial disease, there will be a delay in the restoration of blood flow, but once perfusion is restored, the leg will go a red-orange colour (sometimes described as sunset foot) due to a profound metabolic vasodilatation before returning to normal colour. This is a positive Buerger's sign.

Doppler ultrasonography

This is used to measure flow in peripheral vessels to provide information about the arteries (e.g. in peripheral vascular disease) and the veins (e.g. in suspected deep venous thrombosis). It uses ultrasound, in a similar way to that in echocardiography, to map out the vessel – highlighting any stenosis. Red blood cells move relative to the ultrasound beam. They create a Doppler shift, which is a change in the frequency of the ultrasound echo that returns to the transducer. The shift in frequency is directly proportional to the velocity of the blood. Colour can be used to differentiate blood flowing towards the probe from blood flowing away. It is commonly used to assess peripheral vessel function before a site is selected for angiography.

Doppler can also be used to calculate the ankle–brachial pressure index (ABPI). The Doppler-derived systolic pressure from one of the foot pulses in the ankle (usually the dorsalis pedis) is divided into the Doppler-derived systolic pressure in the brachial artery recorded with the patient lying down (when the pressures should be equal). This ratio provides useful information about the severity of peripheral vascular disease:

- ABPI >0.7 indicates normal vessel calibre (the blood pressure in the feet may be slightly higher than in the arms due to the effect of gravity).
- ABPI <0.7 indicates a degree of peripheral vascular disease (the blood pressure in the feet is less than that in the arm due to atheroma formation or diabetic vessel changes).
- ABPI <0.3 indicates critical ischaemia (the blood pressure in the feet is so low it is likely the patient will be experiencing symptoms of ischaemia at rest).

Aneurysmal disease

An aneurysm is an abnormal, permanent dilatation of an artery or portion of an artery. True aneurysms involve all three layers of the vessel wall and can be classified morphologically as fusiform or saccular (Fig. 9.1). False (or pseudo-) aneurysms occur when blood leaks out of a vessel but is contained by the outer layers of the vessel or surrounding connective tissue. A dissecting aneurysm (or dissection) occurs when there is a tear in the vessel intima that allows blood to flow into the wall, creating an additional channel (the false lumen) between the intima and media through which blood can flow. This intimal tear can result from shear forces acting on the intima from within the vessel lumen or from internal rupture of a small haematoma within the vessel media.

An aneurysm can theoretically develop in any artery; however, they are by far most common in the aorta, in particular, the abdominal aorta where they are a common finding in elderly males. The most common site for a peripheral aneurysm is the popliteal artery. The

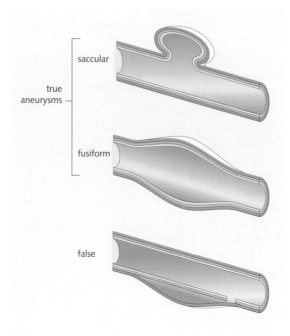

Fig. 9.1 Types of aneurysm: saccular, fusiform, and false.

development of aneurysms can be caused by a number of factors:

- Atherosclerosis: this is the most common cause. The migration of smooth muscle cells from the media into the intimal lesion weakens the wall, promoting aneurysm development. In addition atherosclerosis affecting the vasa vasorum supplying the vessel wall can cause ischaemia/infarction of the wall, weakening it further.
- Cystic medial degeneration: affects the thoracic aorta primarily and predisposes to development of aneurysm and dissection. There is degeneration of the media and reduction in elasticity. This occurs particularly in patients with connective tissue disorders such as Marfan's syndrome.
- Vasculitis: conditions such as Kawasaki's disease (causes coronary artery aneurysms), giant cell arteritis (predisposes to ascending aortic aneurysms) and Takayasu's arteritis all predispose to aneurysm development.
- Infection: tertiary syphilis can lead to the development of saccular aneurysms in the proximal aorta. These are referred to as luetic aneurysms.
- Congenital: small saccular aneurysms in the circle of Willis in the cerebral circulation called Berry aneurysms (Fig. 9.2). If these rupture they cause a subarachnoid haemorrhage.

Aneurysms are often asymptomatic but can cause symptoms following any of the following complications:

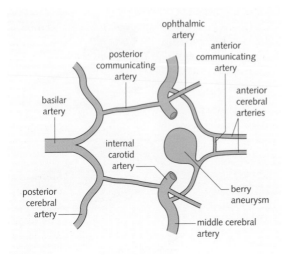

Fig. 9.2 Berry aneurysm in the circle of Willis.

- Rupture: the likelihood of rupture increases with the degree of aneurysmal dilatation. Rupture can cause massive blood loss, particularly in the case of the aorta, which can be rapidly fatal.
- Thrombosis: altered haemodynamics in the aneurysmal segment of vessel can lead to the development of a thrombus within the aneurysm. This thrombus can extend and obstruct the vessel.
- Embolism: small pieces of thrombus can detach from the thrombus lining the aneurysm, which may then occlude distal vessels, causing acute ischaemia. The calibre of vessel occluded depends on the size of the thrombus. Small emboli may lodge in small distal vessels causing digital ischaemia while large emboli may occlude larger vessels causing acute limb ischaemia or acute bowel ischaemia.
- Pressure: as the aneurysm expands it can compress adjacent structures. For example, an aneurysm in the aortic arch can compress the oesophagus causing dysphagia (difficultly swallowing).

Ultrasound scanning is a useful tool for the assessment of peripheral aneurysms, as it allows quantification of the vessel diameter. In the aorta, however, ultrasound scanning gives poor visualization and computed tomography (CT) scanning with intravenous contrast is the investigation of choice. Magnetic resonance imaging (MRI) can also be used to give high-resolution images. A CT scan of an abdominal aortic aneurysm is shown in Fig. 9.3.

Abdominal aortic aneurysm

Abdominal aortic aneurysms are present in approximately 3% of men over 50. They can be asymptomatic and identified incidentally on physical examination with an expansile mass in the abdomen, or during

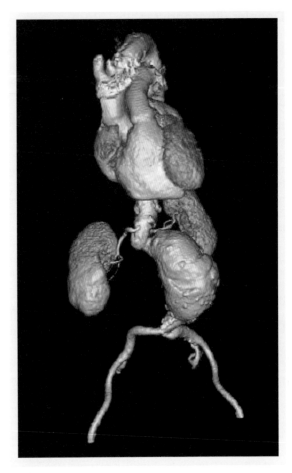

Fig. 9.3 CT of an abdominal aortic aneurysm. (Courtesy of Professor Newby.)

imaging studies for another purpose. Some will present with back pain due to compression of retroperitoneal structures, or abdominal pain. The most feared complication is rupture, which leads to catastrophic blood loss and is associated with very high mortality. The chance of rupture increases with the size of the aneurysm and is increased in hypertensive individuals. Currently, intervention is indicated when the diameter exceeds 5.5 cm or the patient is symptomatic. Treatment options include:

- Surgical: a synthetic graft to replace the aneurysmal segment of the aorta.
- Endovascular: a synthetic graft is introduced percutaneously via the femoral artery and placed in the aneurysmal segment. The aneurysm is then excluded from the aortic blood flow.

Aortic dissection

In aortic dissection, a false lumen is created within the aortic wall as a result of a tear in the intima. It usually occurs in the thoracic aorta due to the high physical forces exerted on the vessel wall. The most widely used classification of aortic dissection is the Stanford classification:

- Type A: involves the ascending aorta.
- Type B: does not involve the ascending aorta.

Aortic dissection is most common in people with hypertension and those with connective tissue disorders such as Marfan's syndrome. Pregnancy is also an important risk factor for aortic dissection. Patients with aortic dissection typically present with severe sudden onset chest pain, sometimes radiating to the back. It is always important to consider this diagnosis in patients presenting with chest pain. Diagnosis is usually made using CT scanning or MRI. A sagittal MRI scan of an aortic dissection is shown in Fig. 9.4.

Sequelae of dissection include:

- Rupture, which is rapidly fatal.
- Occlusion of aortic branches, especially coronary, cerebral, and renal arteries.
- Proximal extension of the dissection can cause aortic regurgitation or cardiac tamponade.

Acute type A dissection has a mortality rate of 1–2% per hour during the first 48 h and a 90% mortality at 30 days if left untreated. Classically, type A dissections (high risk of rupture) are treated surgically by replacing the affected segment of the aorta with a synthetic graft, while type B dissections (which are not as immediately life-threatening) are treated medically with tight blood pressure control to reduce wall stress or with endovascular stenting.

Carotid artery disease

Atherosclerotic plaques commonly develop at the bifurcation of the carotid artery. The consequences of this can cause significant problems:

- Severe, stable stenosis, if occurring bilaterally, can lead to cerebral hypoperfusion causing confusion or syncope.
- Thrombi can form on the surface of the atheroma and throw off small emboli to the cerebral circulation. This can cause an embolic stroke or a transient ischaemic attack (mimics a stroke but symptoms last less than 24 h).

On examination, a carotid bruit (sounds similar to a systolic murmur) may be heard during auscultation of the neck but this is not a reliable sign. This is produced by abnormal turbulent flow that develops as the normal laminar flow is disturbed by the stenosis. Doppler ultrasound can be used to assess the presence and degree of stenosis. Intervention is usually performed in symptomatic patients with a greater than 70% stenosis. Options include carotid endarterectomy, in which surgeons open the carotid artery and scrape out the atheroma or carotid artery stenting to compress the atheroma, increasing vessel patency.

DISEASES OF THE VEINS

The venous system of the lower limbs comprises a deep and a superficial system. Fig. 9.5 depicts the major superficial veins, the long and short saphenous veins. These join the femoral vein and popliteal vein (deep veins) respectively, as well as giving off a number of small perforating veins to the deep veins. Blood flows into the deep veins and with the aid of the skeletal (primarily calf) muscle pump and the numerous valves, the blood is returned to the central veins. There are two important conditions of the veins to understand, varicose veins, which affect the superficial venous system, and deep vein thrombosis, which affects the deep venous system.

Varicose veins

Varicose veins are tortuous, dilated superficial veins, usually of the lower limbs, caused by valvular incompetence. They occur in 10–20% of the normal population, and although far more women present to hospital or

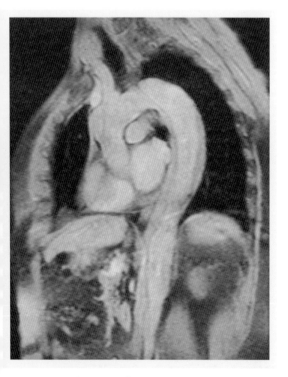

Fig. 9.4 Sagittal MRI scan showing extensive aortic dissection. Note how the descending aorta seems to have two lumens (double-barrelled). (Courtesy of Dr A Timmis and Dr S Brecker.)

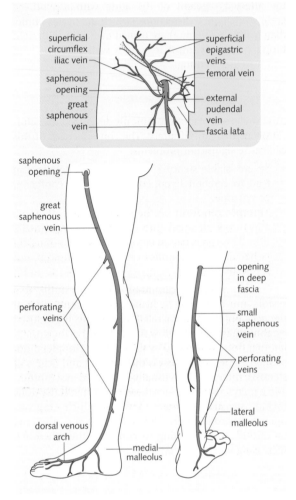

Fig. 9.5 Perforating veins of the lower limbs.

their GP as a result of their varicose veins, the actual incidence is thought to be the same in men and women. Risk factors include:

- Pregnancy.
- Obesity.
- Prolonged standing: therefore it is important to know the patient's occupation.
- Previous deep vein thrombosis.
- Pelvic masses compressing the deep veins.

Aetiology

As discussed above, blood is returned mainly through the deep veins to the thoracic compartment by the skeletal pumping effect of the calf muscles. If there is an obstruction to flow in the deep veins (e.g. by thrombosis or pelvic mass) or there are incompetent valves in the perforating veins, then blood will move from the deep

veins into the superficial veins. This will lead to distension and further valvular incompetence, resulting in stasis of blood. Oedema and skin changes develop, which fail to heal as a result of the impaired circulation.

Sequelae of varicose veins include:

- Bleeding: mild trauma can cause profuse bleeding from varicose veins because pressures are high and the walls of the vein are thin and distended.
- Phlebitis: inflammation of the vessel wall that may be complicated by bacterial infection.
- Venous eczema: skin becomes thin and has a brown discolouration. It is caused by leakage of cells into the tissue due to the high venous pressure, which then break down releasing haemosiderin into the skin.
- Venous ulcers: usually occur on the medial aspect of the lower leg (the gaiter area). They tend to be shallow and often contain pink granulation tissue as they attempt to heal.

Varicose veins do not always require treatment. Occasionally, patients complain of a dragging sensation, bleeding or are disturbed by the appearance of their legs. In these patients, surgery may be appropriate to remove the distended veins.

> **HINTS AND TIPS**
>
> Ulceration often occurs on the lower limbs, and distinguishing between the different causes clinically is often very difficult. Arterial ulcers are usually deep, punched out lesions on the lateral aspect of the foot, between the toes and on pressure points. Venous ulcers are most often sloughy, and on the medial aspect of the calf in the gaiter area. The key to detecting neuropathic ulceration is to test the sensation in the feet. Diabetic ulcers tend to be a mixture of neuropathic and micro-angiopathic ulcers.

> Varicose veins affect a large number of people, those who stand for long periods of time, e.g. teachers, being particularly at risk. Treatment may be conservative, i.e. compression bandaging, or surgical. Surgical treatment may be local, e.g. injection of sclerosant into the dilated vein, or generalized, e.g. tying off the incompetent valve and stripping out the dilated vein.

Other sites of varicosities

Increased venous pressures can cause abnormal dilatation of veins elsewhere in the body. These include:

- Haemorrhoids (piles) are distended submucosal veins in the anal canal that may protrude through the anus. Bleeding and pain may result from trauma, protrusion or spasm of the anal sphincter.
- Varicocoele is a distension of the veins of the pampiniform plexus in the spermatic cord.
- Oesophageal varices are distended veins at the oesophageal–gastric junction. They are caused by portal hypertension, usually as a result of liver cirrhosis.

Deep vein thrombosis (DVT)

DVT describes the presence of a thrombus within the deep veins of the leg and develops most commonly in the deep veins of the thigh or in the deep veins of the calf. Often DVT is asymptomatic but it can cause calf pain, unilateral leg swelling with raised skin temperature and dilated superficial veins. The major concern in a patient with a DVT is that part of the thrombus will detach and embolize to the pulmonary circulation, causing a pulmonary embolism.

Risk factors for thrombosis are used to formulate a Well's score (Fig. 9.6) but can be considered more broadly using Virchow's triad, which describes three prothrombotic conditions:

- Stasis: this can be a result of obstruction to venous outflow from the legs caused by a pelvic mass or by a fetus in a pregnant woman.

- Hypercoagulable state: the oral contraceptive pill and malignancy are both factors that increase the coagulability of the blood.
- Endothelial damage.

> Leg swelling is a result of oedema due to alteration in the forces of fluid filtration. Increased venous pressure will increase the capillary hydrostatic pressure within the leg, increasing fluid filtration and increasing interstitial fluid.

Usually investigation is with Doppler ultrasonography to look for the presence of a thrombus. D-dimers (fibrin degradation products) can also be measured in a patient suspected to have a DVT, but this has poor specificity. As a result, D-dimer measurement is useful for ruling out a DVT but has no role in confirming the diagnosis. The gold standard investigation is venography using intravenous contrast. Initial treatment is anticoagulation with low molecular weight heparin. In patients who suffer a pulmonary embolism and have a persistent DVT, an inferior vena cava (IVC) filter can be considered. As the name suggests, this is a fine filter that is placed in the IVC and prevents emboli from the veins of the leg reaching the pulmonary circulation.

Fig. 9.6 Well's score showing risk factors for deep venous thrombosis (DVT)

Criteria	Score
• Lower limb trauma, surgery, or immobilization in a plaster cast	+1
• Bedridden for more than three days or surgery within last four weeks	+1
• Tenderness along line of femoral or popliteal veins	+1
• Entire limb swollen	+1
• Calf more than 3cm greater in circumference, measured 10 cm below tibial tuberosity	+1
• Pitting oedema	+1
• Dilated collateral superficial veins	+1
• Past history of DVT (confirmed)	+1
• Malignancy	+1
• Intravenous drug use	+3
• Alternative diagnosis more likely than DVT	−2
DVT 'likely' if Well's >1 DVT 'unlikely' if Well's <2	

Basic history and examination of the cardiovascular system

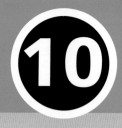

Objectives

You should be able to:
- Understand the important points to note in the cardiovascular history.
- Understand the importance of observing the patient from the end of the bed.
- Recognize clinical signs in the hands and face and know their diagnostic inference.
- Describe how to palpate the peripheral pulses and be aware of abnormalities that may be found.
- Conduct a thorough examination of the thorax including inspection, palpation and auscultation.
- Understand the principles of auscultation of the heart, including valve areas, heart sounds and murmurs.

TAKING A HISTORY

It is not the purpose of this book to discuss the basic principles of taking a medical history, and it will not do so. There are, however, a number of important factors that must be addressed when taking a history of a patient with cardiovascular disease.

As with any history, you should let the patient tell you the natural history of the complaint, but symptoms you should specifically ask about that are relevant to the cardiovascular system include:

- Chest pain.
- Shortness of breath, orthopnoea and paroxysmal nocturnal dyspnoea (PND).
- Oedema/leg swelling.
- Palpitation.
- Syncope (fainting) or dizziness.
- Intermittent claudication.

Risk factors

If the history is consistent with any form of vascular disease (including ischaemic heart disease, peripheral vascular disease and cerebrovascular disease), it is useful to make a list of risk factors for atherosclerosis that the patient does and does not have. See chapter 7 to remind yourself of these. Knowledge of these risk factors helps to formulate a management plan tailored specifically to that individual patient.

Past medical history

Ask the patient if they have any other medical problems and if they have ever undergone a surgical procedure. Important past medical conditions to note include:
- Diabetes mellitus.
- Hypertension.

- Dyslipidaemia/high cholesterol.
- Smoker.
- Myocardial infarction.
- Stroke or transient ischaemic attack.
- Angina.
- Peripheral vascular disease.
- Rheumatic fever.
- Renal disease.

Specific surgical procedures to note include:
- Coronary artery bypass graft (CABG).
- Angioplasty (not strictly surgical, but the patient may see it that way).
- Pacemakers and other implantable devices.
- Vascular surgery.

Family history

Any relevant family history should be noted. Ask whether there is any incidence of the following diseases in close relatives:

- Diabetes mellitus.
- Myocardial infarction.
- Stroke.
- Angina.
- Hypertension.

A positive family history for myocardial infarction is regarded as <55 years for a male first-degree relative and <65 for a female first-degree relative.

Review of systems

Respiratory system

Note the presence of any cough, sputum or haemoptysis, which may occur in a patient with pulmonary oedema. A dry cough is a side-effect of angiotensin-converting enzyme (ACE) inhibitors.

Gastrointestinal system

Abdominal (particularly epigastric) pain might be caused by a myocardial infarction. Other abdominal pain might be caused by an aortic aneurysm or bowel ischaemia due to obstruction of the mesenteric vessels.

Genitourinary system

Cardiovascular causes of increased frequency of micturition and increased urine production include diabetes mellitus and diuretic therapy. Intermittent supraventricular tachycardias may also cause increased urine production. Nocturia (needing to micturate at night) is common in heart failure.

> **HINTS AND TIPS**
>
> When taking a history it is important to individualize it to the patient in order to gain a holistic view. This is particularly important with risk factors for ischaemic heart disease, and how their angina limits their hobbies and activities.

CLINICAL EXAMINATION

This is not an exhaustive account of the clinical signs that may be encountered in patients with cardiovascular disease, but it provides an overview that is sufficient for those in the early stages of clinical training.

Before beginning your examination it is always important to introduce yourself to the patient, gain consent to examine the patient and ensure they are adequately exposed. The patient should be seated at 45° and the whole upper body exposed. Examination should then begin with you standing at the end of the bed and observing the patient.

General appearance

Note the general appearance of the patient. Think about whether the patient looks comfortable or if they are in pain. The patient may be obviously short of breath, look pale or may be cyanosed (blueish tinge to the skin). At this point you should make a note of any oxygen masks or intravenous infusions that the patient is receiving. You may also hear the clicking sound of a mechanical heart valve replacement.

Hands and arms

Both hands should be inspected on the anterior and posterior aspects. Signs that may be present in the hands are shown in Fig. 10.1.

Radial pulse

Palpate the radial pulse with the tips of the fingers and gently compress the radial artery against the head of the radius. The radial pulse is used to assess heart rate and rhythm. The pulse character and volume, however, are best assessed at the carotid artery. The rate should be counted for about 30 seconds and then doubled to give a rate per minute. A normal pulse is between 60 and 100 beats per minute (bpm). Anything outside this range is termed bradycardia (<60 bpm) or tachycardia (>100 bpm). The rhythm may be regular or irregular; if it is irregular, note whether it is a repeating irregularity (regularly irregular) or is completely irregular (irregularly irregular):

- Regular: normal rhythm; remember sinus arrhythmia is normal (an increased rate during inspiration).
- Regularly irregular: commonly caused by ectopic systolic beats or second-degree heart block.
- Irregularly irregular: usually caused by atrial fibrillation, but an ECG is required to confirm this.

Radioradial delay is delay of the left radial pulse compared with the right; this may be due to an aortic dissection affecting the proximal aorta or due to subclavian artery stenosis. Radiofemoral delay is delay of the femoral pulse compared with the radial; this may be due to coarctation of the aorta. Checking for a collapsing pulse (see below) is also often performed at the wrist. The flats of the examiner's fingers should be placed over the radial artery, and the shoulder flexed. A positive result is a bounding pulse, which rapidly falls.

> **HINTS AND TIPS**
>
> Taking the radial pulse affords a good opportunity to observe the patient, and also to measure the respiratory rate. The respiratory rate often rises when patients think it is being measured!

Brachial pulse

Palpate just above the medial aspect of the antecubital fossa and compress the brachial artery against the humerus. If you have trouble, palpate the tendon of biceps and move your fingers medial to it. People will usually assess the brachial pulse OR the carotid pulse for the pulse character.

Blood pressure

A measurement of blood pressure should be taken in all patients. As well as observing whether the blood pressure is high or low, think about whether the pulse

Fig. 10.1 Examination of the hands

Area	Sign observed	Diagnostic inference
Nails	Clubbing (loss of the angle at the base of the nail) 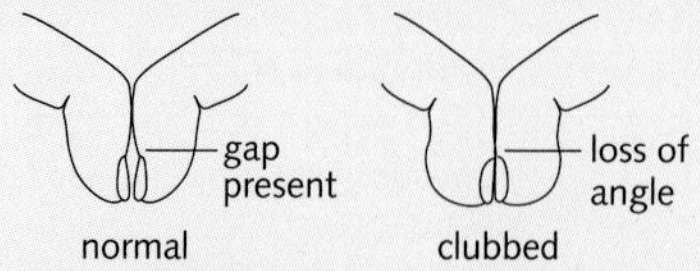 normal clubbed	Infective endocarditis and cyanotic congenital heart disease Other causes: bronchial carcinoma, bronchial empyema/abscess, bronchiectasis, cystic fibrosis, fibrosing alveolitis, mesothelioma, Crohn's disease, cirrhosis, coeliac disease, gastrointestinal lymphoma
	Splinter haemorrhages (small, linear, haemorrhages under the nail that are splinter-like) 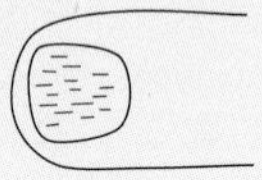	Infective endocarditis; commonly found after trauma to the nail, especially in manual workers
	Tobacco stains	Smoking
Fingers	Osler's nodes (red, painful, transient swellings on pulp of fingers and toes)	Infective endocarditis
Palms	Janeway lesions (small, erythematous macules on the thenar and hypothenar eminences that blanch under pressure)	Infective endocarditis
Dorsum	Tendon xanthomas (yellow nodules over the extensor tendons)	Familial hypercholesterolaemia

Note: finger clubbing is an important sign of disease, and it should always be checked for. Clubbing is demonstrated by abnormal curvature of the nail, fluctuation of the nail bed and loss of the angle between the nail bed and the nail itself.

pressure is normal, increased or decreased. This can give useful clues as to the diagnosis.

Face and neck

Signs that may be found in the face are shown in Fig. 10.2. Examination of the retinas with an ophthalmoscope may reveal evidence of microvascular damage caused by diabetes mellitus or hypertension and may reveal Roth's spots (retinal haemorrhages) in a patient with infective endocarditis. In practice, however, this is not routinely performed.

Carotid pulse

The carotid pulse should be palpated by pressing backwards at the medial border of the sternocleidomastoid and lateral to the thyroid cartilage. The two pulses should never be palpated at the same time or you will risk restricting the cerebral blood supply. The carotid pulse should be used to assess the character of the pulse (Fig. 10.3). This may be difficult, and it is important to note that there are variations of normal pulse character. The important pulses to note are:

- Slow rising pulse: the pulse rises slowly to a peak and then falls slowly. It is of small volume. This suggests aortic stenosis.
- Collapsing (water-hammer) pulse: there is a rapid rise to the pulse and then a rapid fall. It is usually found in aortic regurgitation but may also be found in patent ductus arteriosus.
- Bisferiens pulse: this is a combination of a slow rising and collapsing pulse. It is indicative of aortic stenosis and regurgitation (mixed aortic valve disease).
- Pulsus alternans: this is composed of alternating strong and weak pulses. It indicates severe left ventricular dysfunction.
- Pulsus paradoxus: this is a pulse that is weaker or even disappears on inspiration. Although blood pressure can decrease slightly during inspiration in a normal individual, if it drops by more than 10 mmHg it is defined as pulsus paradoxus and is abnormal. It can occur in cardiac tamponade, constrictive pericarditis or a tension pneumothorax.

Fig. 10.2 Examination of the face*		
Area	**Sign observed**	**Diagnostic inference**
Eyes	Xanthelasma (lipid deposits above or below the eye)	Hypercholesterolaemia
	Conjunctival pallor	Anaemia
	Exophthalmos (protrusion of the eyeballs from their sockets)	Thyrotoxicosis
	Corneal arcus (crescenteric opacity in the periphery of the cornea)	Common in old people; hypercholesterolaemia
Retina	Microaneurysm (small vascular leaks caused by capillary occlusion)	Diabetes mellitus
	Cotton-wool spots (white exudate around the macula)	Hypertension; arterial occlusion; ischaemia of the retina
	Flame-shaped haemorrhages (haemorrhage around optic disc spreading outwards)	Hypertension
	Papilloedema (swelling of the optic nerve head caused by raised intracranial pressure)	Malignant hypertension; chronic meningitis; brain tumour or abscess; subdural haematoma
	Roth's spots	Infective endocarditis
Skin	Malar flush (peripheral cyanosis on cheeks)	Mitral stenosis
Lips and tongue	Central cyanosis	Pulmonary–systemic shunting; lung disease; haemoglobinopathy
Palate	High–arched	Marfan syndrome
Oral cavity	Poor dentition and oral hygeine	May be more prone to infective endocarditis

Generally this is restricted to just inspection unless other systems are also being assessed.

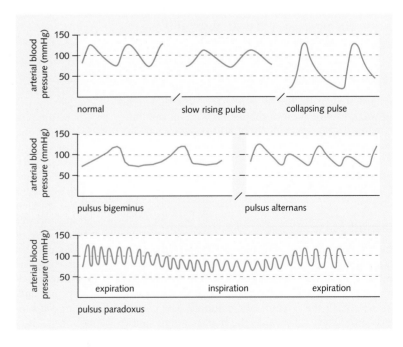

Fig. 10.3 Characters of pulses. The various pulse waveforms that can result are shown here.

The volume of the pulse should also be assessed. A low volume implies a decreased stroke volume. A high volume pulse (sometimes described as bounding) may be caused by conditions including anaemia, carbon dioxide retention, liver disease, sepsis or thyrotoxicosis in which cardiac output is high.

Jugular venous pulse

The internal jugular vein reflects the right atrial pressure. The reasons behind this and the components of the normal waveform are described in Chapter 4. You should observe the maximum height of the jugular venous pulse (JVP) and the character of the pulsation as follows (Fig. 10.4):

1. Place the patient at a 45° angle, with the neck supported to relax the neck muscles. You may need to turn the patient's head away from you slightly.
2. Observe the junction of the sternocleidomastoid with the clavicle and then look up along the route of the jugular veins to see if you can see any visible pulsations.
3. Try palpating the pulse. If you can feel it, then the pulse is probably from the carotid artery. Venous pulses are almost impossible to feel. Furthermore, the venous pulse is usually complex, with two impulses and a dominant inward wave, whereas the arterial pulse is usually a simple dominant outward wave. The jugular venous pulse also decreases with inspiration under normal circumstances.
4. Estimate the vertical height of the pulse from the manubriosternal angle (angle of Louis). This gives an indication of the jugular venous pressure, a direct indicator of right atrial pressure.

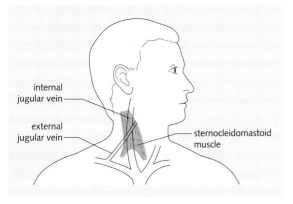

Fig. 10.4   The course of the internal and external jugular veins.

Fig. 10.5 The normal JVP and some common abnormalities (a, a wave; c, c wave; v, v wave; x, x descent; y, y descent).

Abnormality	Diagnostic inference
Dominant a wave	Pulmonary stenosis, pulmonary hypertension, tricuspid stenosis
Canon a wave	Complete beat block, paroxysmal nodal tachycardia, ventricular tachycardia
Dominant v wave	Tricuspid regurgitation
Absent x descent	Atrial fibrillation
Exaggerated x descent	Cardiac tamponade, constrictive pericarditis
Sharp y descent	Constrictive pericarditis, tricuspid regurgitation
Slow y descent	Right atrial myxoma

The external jugular vein is often easier to see, as it is lateral to the sternocleidomastoid and more superficial. However, it is an unreliable indicator of central venous pressure. It contains valves and moves through many fascial planes, and so it is affected by compression from structures in the neck. Some common abnormalities of the JVP waveform are described in Fig. 10.5.

A raised jugular venous pulse (>4 cm above the manubriosternal angle) is usually indicative of:

- Right heart failure.
- Superior vena cava obstruction (this also abolishes any pulsations).
- Intravascular volume overload (e.g. acute nephritis, excess fluid therapy).

If the jugular venous pulse rises on inspiration (Kussmaul's sign) then consider:

- Constrictive pericarditis.
- Cardiac tamponade.
- Tension pneumothorax.

If the jugular venous pulse is not visible, you may attempt to elicit the hepatojugular reflex. This involves applying pressure over the liver, which should increase venous return, raise central venous pressure and cause the jugular venous pressure to rise and become visible. If the jugular venous pulse was originally so high that it was not visible in the neck (i.e. the venous pulse was in the jaw), then this manoeuvre will not elicit any change. Observation of the jugular venous pulse gives a good indication of right atrial pressure and thus right-sided cardiac filling pressures. This can be measured more accurately by the placement of a central line in the internal jugular vein. Normal central venous pressure is 0–10 cmH$_2$O.

Thorax

Inspection

Thorough inspection of the thorax should include asking the patient to lift their arms. Look for scars, chest wall deformities, abnormal pulsations and a pacemaker/implantable cardiac defibrillator implant (usually just below the clavicle on the left). Important scars to be aware of include a median sternotomy, lateral thoracotomy and mitral valvotomy scar (may be hidden under the breast in a female patient).

Palpation

The apex beat should be palpated first. The apex beat is defined as the most inferior-lateral point at which the cardiac impulse can be felt and is normally located in the fifth intercostal space in the mid-clavicular line (Fig. 10.6). If the apex beat is displaced (usually inferolaterally) it indicates cardiac dilatation. In left ventricular hypertrophy, due to hypertension or aortic stenosis for example, the apex beat is more forceful. It is important to remember the distinction between ventricular dilatation (which causes displacement of the apex beat) and hypertrophy (which increases the force of the apex beat). The left sternal edge should be palpated with the

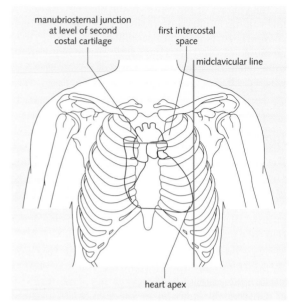

Fig. 10.6 Position of the apex beat. The apex beat is the position most inferior and furthest lateral that the cardiac impulse can be felt. As a guide to identifying intercostal spaces, the second rib lies lateral to the manubriosternal angle; the second intercostal space is below this rib. The lateral position can also be described relative to the anterior axillary line and the mid-axillary line. The normal apex beat lies in the fifth intercostal space, mid-clavicular line.

palm of the hand for a right ventricular heave and finally, all four valve areas (see below) should be palpated with the lateral border of the hand for a thrill.

Auscultation

The stethoscope has two ends, the bell and the diaphragm (this is the larger, flatter end). The diaphragm is better for listening to higher pitched sounds; therefore, it is best for hearing:

- First and second heart sounds.
- Third and fourth heart sounds.
- Systolic murmurs.
- Aortic diastolic murmurs (aortic incompetence).

Finally, use the diaphragm to auscultate the bases of the lungs to check for signs of pulmonary oedema (i.e. fine crackles) or pleural effusion (absent breath sounds).

Normal heart sounds

Initially, concentrate on identifying the normal heart sounds first – a repetitive 'lupp-dubb'. Auscultating while palpating the carotid pulse will help to distinguish the heart sounds. The first heart sound (S_1) coincides with the onset of systole and, therefore, the carotid pulse. The second heart sound (S_2) coincides with the beginning of diastole. Occasionally, the heart sounds may be split, when one component of the sound occurs before the other. S_2 is normally split on inspiration, especially in the young. The heart sounds have already been discussed in Chapter 4.

Added heart sounds

The third and fourth heart sounds (S_3 and S_4, respectively) occur in diastole. S_3 is sometimes heard in healthy, young adults (younger than 35 years) and in pregnant women. Otherwise, the presence of S_3 suggests:

- Heart failure.
- Mitral regurgitation.
- High-cardiac output states.

The presence of S_4 indicates a ventricle with decreased compliance (e.g. due to aortic stenosis or hypertension when the ventricle becomes hypertrophied).

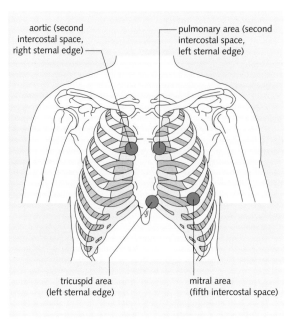

aortic (second intercostal space, right sternal edge)

pulmonary area (second intercostal space, left sternal edge)

tricuspid area (left sternal edge)

mitral area (fifth intercostal space)

Fig. 10.7 Auscultatory areas. This shows where the valve sounds are best heard. These areas are not the surface markings of where the valves actually are.

The bell of the stethoscope is best for low-pitched sounds and is best for hearing the rumbling diastolic murmur of mitral stenosis. The bell should not be placed too tightly to the skin, as it will then function as a diaphragm.

There are certain areas where auscultation should be performed (Fig. 10.7); these are the areas where murmurs from heart valves are best heard:

- Mitral area: fifth intercostal space, mid-clavicular line.
- Tricuspid area: fourth intercostal space, left sternal edge.
- Aortic area: second intercostal space, right sternal edge.
- Pulmonary area: second intercostal space, left sternal edge.

If a systolic murmur is heard, the axilla and the carotid arteries should be auscultated with the diaphragm of the stethoscope for radiation. The murmur of mitral regurgitation often radiates to the axilla and the murmur of aortic stenosis classically radiates to the carotid arteries, although it can also sometimes be heard in the axilla.

Diastolic murmurs can be quiet and difficult to hear. Rolling the patient onto their left-hand side brings the apex of the heart into contact with the chest wall and may make the murmur of mitral stenosis audible. By asking the patient to sit forward and hold their breath in expiration, a murmur of aortic regurgitation can be heard better at the left sternal edge.

> ### HINTS AND TIPS
>
> S_3 can be benign or pathological but S_4 is always pathological.

Alterations in sound intensity can indicate disease, for example:

- S_1 is loud in mitral stenosis and soft in mitral regurgitation.
- S_2 is loud in hypertension and soft in aortic stenosis.

Murmurs

Murmurs are caused by turbulent blood flow at a valve or an abnormal communication within the heart. The presence of a murmur does not always indicate disease, and the loudness does not correlate with the severity of the lesion. The common murmurs that you are likely to encounter are shown in Fig. 10.8. Many individuals have benign, innocent murmurs, called flow murmurs. These typically:

- Are soft, early systolic murmurs.
- Occur in the young or the elderly.
- Occur in conditions with increased cardiac output (e.g. anaemia, thyrotoxicosis, hypertension, pregnancy).

Fig. 10.8 The common types of cardiac murmur

Timing	Cause	Best heard	Radiates
Systolic murmurs: Ejection systolic S_1 S_2 S_1	Aortic stenosis Pulmonary stenosis	Aortic area Left sternal edge	Neck Loudest on inspiration
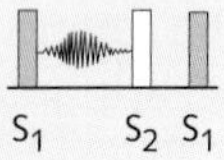 Pansystolic S_1 S_2 S_1	Mitral regurgitation (blowing) Tricuspid regurgitation (low-pitched) Ventricular septal defect (loud and rough)	Apex Left sternal edge Left sternal edge	Axilla – –
Diastolic murmurs: Mid-diastolic S_1 S_2 S_1	Mitral stenosis (low rumbling) Tricuspid stenosis	Apex Left sternal edge	Louder with exercise –
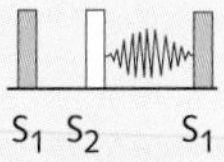 Early diastolic S_1 S_2 S_1	Aortic regurgitation (blowing, high-pitched) Pulmonary regurgitation	Left sternal edge Right sternal edge	– –
Continuous murmurs: S_1 S_2 S_1 Combined systolic and diastolic murmurs	Patent ductus arteriosus (machinery) Aortic stenosis and regurgitation	Left sternal edge Left sternal edge	– Neck

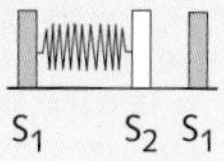

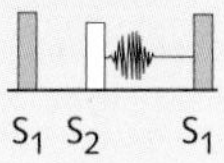

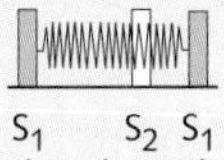

When describing a murmur you should consider the following:

- Systolic or diastolic?
- The character of the murmur.
- Where is it heard loudest?
- Does it radiate?

Abdomen

If there are any signs of heart failure, it may be useful to palpate the liver. An enlarged liver can occur due to venous congestion in heart failure affecting the right ventricle. In tricuspid regurgitation, the liver may be pulsatile.

The abdominal aorta should also be palpated. This is performed by placing two hands on the abdomen around the level of the umbilicus and feeling for the pulsatile aorta. If it is aneurysmal it will be expansile, i.e. push your hands apart.

Legs

It is important to always check the ankles for pitting oedema, which is a sign of heart failure. Gently press on the skin over a bony landmark such as the medial malleolus, and if pitting oedema is present, an imprint of your finger will be left after you remove it. You should comment on whether it is unilateral or bilateral and how far it extends up the legs. In patients who are in bed, sacral oedema may develop, so it is often useful to check for that while the patient is leaning forward for you to auscultate to their lung bases.

Finally, you should palpate all the peripheral pulses, as described in Chapter 9.

Cardiovascular examination summary

See Fig. 10.9.

Fig. 10.9 Template for examination of the cardiovascular system

introduce, consent and expose the patient general inspection	
Hands	clubbing, peripheral cyanosis, nicotine staining, splinter haemorrhages, Janeway lesions, Osler's nodes.
Radial pulse	rate, rhythm, volume
Blood pressure	
Face	corneal arcus, malar flush, conjunctival pallor, xanthelasma, central cyanosis
JVP	height and waveform
Carotid pulse	character, volume
Thorax inspection	scars, deformity, pulsation
Thorax palpation	apex beat position and character, left parasternal heave, thrills
Auscultation	mitral area (bell and diaphragm)
	tricuspid area
	pulmonary area
	aortic area
	axilla and carotid artery
	lung bases
Abdomen	palpate the liver
Legs	ankle oedema
	peripheral pulses

Note: all of these points should be considered in a thorough cardiovascular examination, as will be expected in an OSCE exam.

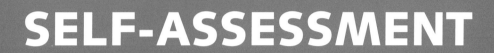

SELF-ASSESSMENT

Single best answer questions (SBAs)

Chapter 2 Anatomy, histology and development of the cardiovascular system

1. Which of the following is not contained within the mediastinum?
   a. The heart.
   b. The lungs.
   c. The thymus gland.
   d. The root of the aorta.
   e. The pulmonary veins.

2. In a normal heart which of the following valves has two cusps?
   a. Aortic.
   b. Pulmonary.
   c. Mitral.
   d. Tricuspid.
   e. All of the above.

3. Which of the following statements regarding cardiac myocytes is true?
   a. They are multinucleated.
   b. They are longer than skeletal muscle fibres.
   c. They never have the ability to generate a spontaneous action potential.
   d. Force of contraction is determined solely by the degree to which cytoplasmic Ca^{2+} increases.
   e. They have a branched structure.

4. Which of the following regarding the coronary vessels is false?
   a. The coronary arteries arise from the aorta just distal to the aortic valve.
   b. The left coronary artery gives rise to a circumflex branch.
   c. The right coronary artery gives rise to the posterior descending artery.
   d. Blood from the coronary veins drains into the coronary sinus and then into the right atrium.
   e. In the majority of people the SA node and AV node are supplied with blood from the left coronary artery.

5. Which of the following congenital heart defects causes cyanosis early in life?
   a. Coarctation of the aorta.
   b. Ventricular septal defect.
   c. Tetralogy of Fallot.
   d. Atrial septal defect.
   e. None of the above.

6. Which of the following does not occur after birth?
   a. There is an increase in pulmonary vascular resistance.
   b. Blood flow through the umbilical vessels decreases.
   c. The foramen ovale between the two atria closes.
   d. The ductus arteriosus closes and becomes the ligamentum arteriosum.
   e. Fetal haemoglobin continues to be produced for around 6 months.

7. What is the second branch of the aorta (excluding the coronary arteries)?
   a. Superior mesenteric artery.
   b. Left common carotid artery.
   c. Right common carotid artery.
   d. Brachiocephalic trunk.
   e. Left subclavian artery.

8. What is the most common congenital heart defect?
   a. Patent ductus arteriosus.
   b. Atrial septal defect.
   c. Bicuspid aortic valve.
   d. Ebstein's anomaly.
   e. Tetralogy of Fallot.

9. Concerning the arteries of the head and neck, which of the following is false?
   a. The circle of Willis is a complete circle.
   b. The ophthalmic artery is a division of the internal carotid artery.
   c. The external jugular vein joins the internal jugular vein on its return to the heart.
   d. The facial artery is a branch of the internal carotid artery.
   e. The veins of the head and neck eventually drain into the superior vena cava.

Chapter 3 Cardiac electrophysiology and arrhythmia

10. In a healthy heart which of the following initiates a heartbeat?
    a. Atrioventricular node.
    b. The left anterior hemifascicle.
    c. The bundle of His.
    d. The sinoatrial node.
    e. The brainstem.

11. On an ECG, the Q–T interval represents the time from:
    a. Atrial depolarization to ventricular repolarization.
    b. Atrial depolarization to ventricular depolarization.

129

c. Ventricular depolarization to ventricular repolarization.
d. Atrial systole to the end of ventricular systole.
e. Atrial depolarization to atrial repolarization.

12. A normal P–R interval should be between:
a. 80 and 200 milliseconds.
b. 120 and 200 milliseconds.
c. 100 and 280 milliseconds.
d. 300 and 500 milliseconds.
e. 500 and 700 milliseconds.

13. Which phase of the cardiac action potential is the major difference between that of cardiomyocytes and skeletal muscle myocytes?
a. 1.
b. 2.
c. 3.
d. 4.
e. 0.

14. The conduction velocity of an action potential is slowest in which of the following?
a. Atrial myocytes.
b. AV nodal myocytes.
c. Bundle of His.
d. Purkinje fibres.
e. Ventricular myocytes.

15. When lying supine, the pressure difference is greatest between which of the following?
a. Portal vein and right atrium.
b. Femoral artery and great saphenous vein.
c. Pulmonary artery and pulmonary vein.
d. Portal vein and hepatic vein.
e. Afferent renal arterioles and efferent renal arteriole.

16. Concerning atrial fibrillation, which of the following statements is false?
a. Alcohol may predispose to this arrhythmia.
b. The atrial component of ventricular filling is lost.
c. All patients with atrial fibrillation require anticoagulation with warfarin.
d. There are no P waves present on the electrocardiogram.
e. Treatment may include DC cardioversion.

17. A ventricular rather than a supraventricular tachycardia is suggested by which of the following?
a. A ventricular rate of >160 beats per minute.
b. Termination of arrhythmia with carotid sinus pressure.
c. A normal cardiac output.
d. An irregularly irregular pulse.
e. QRS complexes >120 ms on an electrocardiogram.

18. On the ECG of a patient with a normal cardiac axis, which of the following leads will have a predominant downward deflection?
a. Lead I.

b. Lead II.
c. AvR.
d. AvF.
e. Chest lead 4.

19. A 68-year-old man presents to his GP for a routine check-up. He is found to have a regularly irregular pulse at a rate of 60 beats per minute. An ECG is performed and shows a normal P–R interval with absence of a QRS complex after every fourth P wave. Which of the following best describes this arrhythmia?
a. Complete heart block.
b. First-degree heart block.
c. Sinus bradycardia.
d. Mobitz type II second-degree heart block.
e. Atrial fibrillation.

Chapter 4 The cardiac cycle and control of cardiac output

20. The pressure wave created by ventricular ejection depends upon all of the following factors except:
a. Stroke volume.
b. Heart rate.
c. Elasticity of the arterial wall.
d. Peripheral vascular resistance.
e. Pulmonary artery pressure.

21. Which of the following statements is correct?
a. Cardiac output is the product of heart rate and end-diastolic volume.
b. Contractility is defined as the force of contraction for a given fibre length.
c. The relationship between end-diastolic volume and end-diastolic pressure is always linear.
d. An increase in contractility causes a downward shift of the Starling curve.
e. Levosimendan exerts its positive inotropic effect by increasing cytosolic Ca^{2+}.

22. Which of the following statements regarding endocarditis is false?
a. Diagnosis is based on the Duke criteria.
b. May occur after dental treatment.
c. Is more common in IV drug users.
d. Can only occur if a bacteraemia is present.
e. Can result in peripheral emboli.

23. In a normal heart, which of the following is true?
a. Right ventricular contraction precedes left ventricular contraction.
b. The c wave of the JVP occurs coincides with the peak velocity of ventricular ejection.
c. Right atrial contraction and left atrial contraction occur simultaneously.

d. During inspiration, the aortic valve closes after the pulmonary valve.

e. The v wave of the JVP coincides with termination of atrial systole.

24. Which of the following does not usually cause an increase in pulse pressure?
   a. Decreased heart rate.
   b. Increasing age.
   c. Septic shock.
   d. Increased left ventricular end-diastolic volume.
   e. Increase in aortic compliance.

25. Which of the following valve lesions is most likely to result from chronic rheumatic heart disease?
   a. Aortic stenosis.
   b. Aortic regurgitation.
   c. Mitral stenosis.
   d. Mitral regurgitation.
   e. Tricuspid regurgitation.

Chapter 5 Haemodynamics and vascular function

26. A 53-year-old Caucasian man has a blood pressure measurement of 162/104 and the GP decides that he should be started on antihypertensive medication. Three weeks later, blood tests reveal that his creatinine has doubled (indicating impaired renal function) and subsequent investigation reveals bilateral renal artery stenosis. What drug was the class of drug the GP prescribed initially?
   a. Beta-blocker.
   b. Ca^{2+} antagonist.
   c. ACE inhibitor.
   d. Thiazide diuretic.
   e. Alpha-blocker.

27. Which of the following organs receives the greatest blood flow per gram of tissue at rest?
   a. Brain.
   b. Liver.
   c. Heart.
   d. Kidney.
   e. Skeletal muscle.

28. According to Poiseuille's law, which of the following does not influence flow in vessels?
   a. Vessel length.
   b. Perfusion pressure.
   c. Blood volume.
   d. Vessel radius.
   e. Blood viscosity.

29. During dynamic exercise, blood flow to active skeletal muscle increases. What is the process that underpins this increase in blood flow?
   a. The exercise reflex.
   b. Functional hyperaemia.

c. Autoregulation.
d. Reactive hyperaemia.
e. The baroreceptor reflex.

30. Regarding flow through the vessels, which of the following is incorrect?
   a. Varies with the pressure difference between one end and the other.
   b. Is directly proportional to the square of the radius.
   c. Decreases directly with the length of the vessel.
   d. Varies inversely with the viscosity of the blood.
   e. Is directly proportional to the velocity of the blood.

31. In the cutaneous circulation, which of the following changes are most likely to occur in response to a decrease in ambient temperature?
   a. Arteriolar vasodilatation.
   b. Relaxation of smooth muscle of arteriovenous anastamoses.
   c. Recruitment of additional capillary units.
   d. Increased perspiration.
   e. Decreased tissue oncotic pressure.

32. Which of the following is true of the renin–angiotensin system (RAS)?
   a. Renin is secreted from the macula densa.
   b. Persistent inhibition of the RAS plays a role in the pathogenesis of heart failure.
   c. Activation of the RAS causes increased excretion of sodium and water from the kidneys.
   d. Angiotensin II brings about vasoconstriction by acting directly on vascular smooth muscle cells.
   e. Angiotensin I is a weak vasodilator.

Chapter 6 Integrated control of the cardiovascular system and cardiovascular reflexes

33. Regarding hormonal control of the cardiovascular system, which of the following statements is correct?
   a. Adrenaline is secreted from the adrenal cortex.
   b. Renin is converted to angiotensin I by angiotensinogen.
   c. ACE is predominately found in the vascular bed of the gastrointestinal tract.
   d. ADH is released when a rise in osmolarity is detected.
   e. Adrenaline/epinephrine causes vasodilatation in skeletal muscle by acting on β_1 receptors.

34. Which of the following does not usually occur in haemorrhagic shock?
   a. Decreased urinary output.
   b. Sweating.
   c. Thirst.
   d. Cutaneous vasoconstriction.
   e. Bradycardia.

35. Which of the following is not a feature of the immediate response to acute haemorrhage:
    a. Total peripheral resistance increases.
    b. Erythropoietin production increases.
    c. Cutaneous arterioles constrict.
    d. Baroreceptor firing decreases.
    e. Release of catecholamines.

36. Which of the following is true of the baroreceptor reflex?
    a. It is central to the long-term regulation of blood pressure.
    b. Decreased loading of baroreceptors increases venous tone by reducing parasympathetic activity.
    c. Constriction of cutaneous arterioles brought about by the baroreceptor reflex can be overcome by thermoregulatory changes in vascular tone.
    d. Baroreceptors in the carotid body are innervated by the glossopharyngeal nerve.
    e. Increased stretch in the arterial wall causes a decrease in baroreceptor firing.

37. Which of the following is responsible for regulation of parasympathetic outflow via the vagus nerve?
    a. Nucleus ambiguus.
    b. Hypothalamic depressor area.
    c. Rostral ventrolateral medulla.
    d. Nucleus tractus solitarius.
    e. Lateral hippocampus.

38. Upon moving from a supine position to standing, which of the following does not usually occur?
    a. There is a decrease in apparent circulating volume due to venous pooling of blood.
    b. Fluid filtration from the interstitium into capillaries increases.
    c. There is a baroreceptor mediated increase in total peripheral resistance.
    d. There is decreased loading of arterial baroreceptors.
    e. Activation of renin secretion.

39. Which of the following cardiovascular reflexes results in an increased parasympathetic outflow and can be used to terminate supraventricular arrhythmias?
    a. Hepatojugular reflex.
    b. Exercise reflex.
    c. Alerting response.
    d. Chemoreceptor reflex.
    e. Diving reflex.

40. During dynamic exercise, which of the following does not occur?
    a. An increase in both systolic and diastolic blood pressure.
    b. An increase in mean arterial blood pressure.
    c. Increased sympathetic outflow to the gastrointestinal, splenic and skeletal muscle vasculature.

    d. Vasodilatation in active muscles causes perfusion of additional capillary units.
    e. Venous return increases in part due to the action of the skeletal muscle pump.

41. During a Valsalva manoeuvre, which of the following is indicative of baroreceptor dysfunction?
    a. An initial increase in arterial blood pressure during stage 1.
    b. Bradycardia during stage 2.
    c. A decrease in blood pressure during stage 3.
    d. Bradycardia during stage 4.
    e. A transient decrease in blood pressure at the beginning of stage 2.

Chapter 7 Atherosclerosis and ischaemic heart disease

42. Which of the flowing cell types are not usually involved in the development of atherosclerosis?
    a. B lymphocytes.
    b. Macrophages.
    c. Smooth muscle cells.
    d. T lymphocytes.
    e. Endothelial cells.

43. A 62-year-old man with a history of hypertension, type 2 diabetes and intermittent claudication presents to A&E with a 1-hour history of crushing central chest pain. An ECG shows ST segment elevation in the anterior leads. Which of the following is likely to be responsible?
    a. Complete occlusion of the left anterior descending artery following rupture of an atherosclerotic plaque.
    b. 30% stenosis of the left main coronary artery by a stable atherosclerotic plaque.
    c. Complete occlusion of the right coronary artery following rupture of an atherosclerotic plaque.
    d. Profound hypoglycaemia.
    e. Severe anaemia.

44. Which of the following statements regarding cardiac enzymes/biomarkers is incorrect?
    a. A raised troponin T level is always due to myocardial infarction.
    b. A negative troponin T at the time of presentation and 12 hours later excludes myocardial infarction.
    c. Lactate dehydrogenase can be elevated following myocardial infarction.
    d. Creatine kinase and troponin I are not raised in unstable angina.
    e. Troponins are a component of myocyte contractile apparatus.

45. Which of the following drugs should not be used in the management of non ST segment elevation myocardial infarction?
    a. Beta-blocker.
    b. Thienopyridine derivative.

c. Recombinant tissue plasminogen activator.
d. Aspirin.
e. Glyceryl trinitrate.

46. A 56-year-old man with a history of hypertension is complaining of central chest pain on exertion that resolves with rest. He is currently taking an ACE inhibitor for his hypertension and a salbutamol inhaler for asthma. His doctor makes a diagnosis of angina pectoris and wants to start him on a drug with negative chronotropic and negative inotropic effects. What would be the most appropriate drug with these actions for this patient?
a. GTN.
b. Verapamil.
c. Amlodipine.
d. Atenolol.
e. Isosorbide mononitrate.

47. Atherosclerosis is best described by which of the following?
a. Inflammatory disease.
b. Degenerative disease.
c. Neoplastic disease.
d. Autoimmune disease.
e. Iatrogenic disease.

48. What is the gold standard investigation for assessing coronary artery disease?
a. Dobutamine stress echocardiogram.
b. CT coronary angiogram.
c. Coronary angiography.
d. Exercise tolerance test.
e. Electrocardiogram.

Chapter 8 Heart failure, myocardial and pericardial disease

49. Which of the following symptoms or signs would you not expect to be present in isolated left ventricular heart failure?
a. Fatigue.
b. Exertional dyspnoea.
c. Orthopnoea.
d. Hepatomegaly.
e. Paroxysmal nocturnal dyspnoea.

50. What is the most common cause of heart failure in the western world?
a. Valvular heart disease.
b. Ischaemic heart disease.
c. Cardiomyopathy.
d. Myocarditis.
e. Hypertension.

51. Which of the following classes of drug are not routinely used in the treatment of chronic heart failure?
a. Beta-blockers.
b. Aldosterone antagonists.

c. Non-dihydropiridine Ca^{2+} channel blockers.
d. ACE inhibitors.
e. Digoxin.

52. Which of the following can not be assessed using transthoracic echocardiography in a patient with heart failure?
a. Ejection fraction.
b. Degree of aortic valve stenosis.
c. Left ventricular wall motion.
d. Left ventricular end-diastolic pressure.
e. Severity of mitral valve regurgitation.

53. What is the most appropriate treatment from the list below for a patient diagnosed with acute pericarditis?
a. Oral beta-blocker.
b. Oral digoxin.
c. IV antibiotics.
d. IV antiviral (e.g. aciclovir).
e. Oral non-steroidal anti-inflammatory.

Chapter 9 Vascular disease

54. The following are features of peripheral vascular disease except:
a. An ankle brachial pressure index greater than 1.
b. Absent foot pulses.
c. Ulceration on the heel of the foot.
d. Intermittent claudication.
e. Shiny, hairless skin.

55. Which of the following has the greatest association with syphilis?
a. Type B aortic dissection.
b. Fusiform popliteal artery aneurysm.
c. Saccular aortic aneurysm.
d. Type A aortic dissection.
e. Penetration atherosclerotic ulcer.

56. Concerning varicose veins, which of the following is true?
a. These are dilated, tortuous deep veins.
b. Immobility and lying flat are strong risk factors.
c. They often occur as a sequelae of deep vein thrombosis.
d. They must always be treated to prevent complications.
e. Histologically, the wall becomes thickened.

57. Which of the following is not a risk factor for deep vein thrombosis?
a. Malignancy.
b. Pregnancy.
c. Family history.
d. Christmas disease.
e. Factor V Leiden deficiency.

58. In a patient with a suspected deep vein thrombosis, what is the most appropriate first line investigation useful for ruling out the diagnosis?
a. D-dimer measurement.
b. CT scan.
c. Serum fibrinogen measurement.
d. Magnetic resonance imaging.
e. Venogram.

59. Which of the following signs and symptoms are caused by acute lower limb ischaemia?
a. Pain.
b. Ulceration.
c. Cold to touch.
d. Weak pulse.
e. Paraesthesia.

60. What is the most common cause of aneurysms?
a. Vasculitis.
b. Infection.
c. Cystic medial degeneration.
d. Atherosclerosis.
e. Iatrogenic.

Chapter 10 Basic history and examination of the cardiovascular system

61. Which of the following are not correct associations?
a. Reverse splitting of the second heart sound – atrial septal defect.
b. Pansystolic murmur – mitral regurgitation.
c. Ejection systolic – pulmonary stenosis.
d. Mid-diastolic murmur – tricuspid stenosis.
e. Continuous murmur – patent ductus arteriosus.

62. Correct findings on auscultation include all of the following except:
a. The first heart sound immediately follows the carotid pulse upstroke.
b. Inspiration causes physiological splitting of the second heart sound.
c. The murmur of aortic stenosis predominantly radiates to the neck.
d. The fourth heart sound, if present, coincides with atrial systole.
e. A mid-systolic click is consistent with mitral valve prolapse.

63. Regarding the character of the pulse, which of the following statements is correct?
a. Aortic regurgitation is associated with a slow rising pulse.
b. A patient with severe restrictive cardiomyopathy may exhibit pulsus paradoxicus.
c. The character of the pulse can be accurately assessed at the radial pulse.
d. Bisferiens pulse has two prominent upstrokes.
e. A collapsing pulse is sometimes referred to as an anacrotic pulse.

64. Which of the following is true when examining the jugular venous pressure?
a. The height of the JVP above the manubriosternal angle gives an estimate of right atrial pressure in mmHg.
b. The patient should be lying flat with their head turned slightly away from the examiner.
c. Gentle pressure over the abdomen elicits the hepatojugular reflex and causes a transient increase in the JVP.
d. The internal jugular vein should be visualized and is usually located just lateral to the sternocleidomastoid.
e. A JVP with a vertical height greater than 2 cm above the manubriosternal angle is abnormal.

Extended matching questions (EMQs)

1. Structure and function of the heart

a. Aorta.

b. Inferior vena cava.

c. Portal vein.

d. Femoral artery.

e. Superior mesenteric artery.

f. Common hepatic artery.

g. Common mesenteric vein.

h. Left renal vein.

i. Inferior mesenteric vein.

j. Azygous vein.

Which one of the structures above best matches each of the descriptions below?

1. Drains the superior and inferior mesenteric veins and the splenic vein.

2. A large elastic artery that gives off the coeliac trunk and renal arteries.

3. Drains the left testicular vein.

2. Cardiac electrophysiology and arrhythmia

a. L-type Ca^{2+} channels.

b. ATP gated K^+ channels.

c. Na^+/Ca^{2+} exchanger.

d. Na^+/K^+ATPase.

e. Voltage gated Na^+ channels.

f. Sarcoplasmic reticulum Ca^{2+}ATPase.

g. Ligand gated membrane Ca^{2+} channel.

h. Intercellular gap junction.

For each description below, select the most appropriate answer from the list above. Each answer may be used once, twice or not at all.

1. Responsible for phase 0 of the fast cell action potential.

2. Responsible for the maintenance of membrane potential during the plateau phase in the fast action potential.

3. Acts to bring about relaxation of cardiomyocytes and removes the majority of the Ca2+ from the cytosol.

4. Blocked by class 1 antiarrhythmic agents.

5. Inhibited by digoxin.

3. Vascular function

a. Increased arterial hydrostatic pressure.

b. Decreased arterial hydrostatic pressure.

c. Increased venous hydrostatic pressure.

d. Decreased venous hydrostatic pressure.

e. Increased interstitial hydrostatic pressure.

f. Decreased interstitial hydrostatic pressure.

g. Increased plasma oncotic pressure.

h. Decreased plasma oncotic pressure.

i. Increased interstitial oncotic pressure.

j. Decreased interstitial oncotic pressure.

Which of these alterations in Starling's forces of capillary fluid filtration occurs in the following situations?

1. A patient with chronic liver disease is found to have swollen ankles and hypoalbuminaemia.

2. A patient with left ventricular failure is short of breath and on examination has bi-basal crackles.

3. A patient with heart failure and swollen ankles starts wearing tight compression stockings and his leg swelling is reduced.

4. Vascular function

a. Nitric oxide.

b. VIP.

c. Substance P.

d. Prostacyclin.

e. Cyclooxygenase.

f. Thromboxane A_2.

g. GMP.

h. Noradrenaline/norepinephrine.

i. Adrenaline/epinephrine.

j. cAMP.

k. Leukotriene.

l. Acetylcholine.

Which of the above best matches the following descriptions?

1. The primary neurotransmitter involved in sympathetic stimulation of vascular smooth muscle.

2. Synthesized and released by endothelial cells and activates soluble guanylyl cyclase in vascular smooth muscle cells.

3. Responsible for production of prostanoids and thromboxanes.

5. Heart failure, myocardial and pericardial disease (this is not specific to Chapter 8)

a. Nifedipine.

b. GTN.

c. Levosimendan.

d. Dobutamine.

e. Adrenaline/epinephrine.

f. Atenolol.

g. Simvastatin.

h. Verapamil.

i. Diltiazem.

j. Lisinopril.

k. Losartan.

l. Digoxin.

m. Spironolactone.

n. Noradrenaline/norepinephrine.

From the list above, pick the drug or class of drug that best fits with the mechanism of action described.

1. Primarily a venodilator but does have some coronary vasodilator effect at higher doses.

2. Acts by inhibiting L-type Ca^{2+} channels in the myocardium, slowing heart rate and reducing contractility.

3. Increases contractility by increasing sensitivity of the contractile apparatus to Ca^{2+}.

6. History and examination

a. Aortic area.

b. Pulmonary area.

c. Mitral area.

d. Tricuspid area.

e. Axilla.

f. Left sternal border.

g. Right sternal border.

h. Weak radial artery pulse.

i. Weak carotid artery pulse.

j. Weak femoral artery pulse.

k. Pansystolic murmur.

l. Continuous murmur.

m. Ejection systolic murmur.

n. Late diastolic murmur.

o. Early diastolic murmur.

Please answer each of the questions below using one of the options listed above.

1. A 67-year-old woman becomes extremely short of breath 3 days after a large myocardial infarction. Doctors suspect that she has ruptured the papillary muscles in the left ventricle. A loud murmur is heard throughout the chest. What is the most likely character of this murmur?

2. A child presents to his GP with pain in both legs when he runs. He is found to have a blood pressure of 176/104. Which of the clinical signs is most likely to be present on examination?

3. The murmur of aortic regurgitation is best heard with the patient leaning forward at end expiration. Where on the chest should a stethoscope be placed to best hear this murmur?

Objective structured clinical examination (OSCE) stations

1. This gentleman has been complaining of shortness of breath on exertion. Please examine his cardiovascular system . . .

Checklist

- Introduce yourself, obtain consent and expose patient from the waist up.
- Observe the patient as a whole from the end of the bed.
- Examine the hands for splinter haemorrhages, clubbing, Osler's nodes, peripheral cyanosis.
- Palpate the radial pulse and comment on the rate and rhythm. Check for radioradial delay.
- State that you would like to measure the patient's blood pressure.
- Inspect the eyes, cheeks and mouth.
- Visualize the jugular venous pressure pulse and comment on its height.
- Palpate the carotid pulse and comment on the character and volume of the pulse.
- Inspect the precordium looking for scars, pacemakers, visual impulses.
- Palpate for the apex beat, heaves and thrills over the valve areas.
- Auscultate the four valve areas, the axilla, neck and lung bases.
- Auscultate for diastolic murmurs; left lateral and sitting forward in held expiration.
- Feel for sacral oedema and pedal oedema.
- Thank the patient and cover him up.

To finish your examination, state that you would like to palpate all peripheral pulses, check for radiofemoral delay, perform fundoscopy and order an ECG.

2. Mr Smith has been suffering from chest pain on exertion for the last 6 months. His general practitioner has told him that he has angina and prescribed him a spray that he is instructed to spray under his tongue when he gets chest pain. Explain to Mr Smith what angina is and the principles of treating it

Checklist

- Angina is a result of inadequate blood supply to the heart when demand is increased such as during exercise.
- It is usually caused by a narrowing of the arteries supplying the heart muscle.
- Management of risk factors such as hypertension, hyperlipidaemia and diabetes is important.
- Patients should stop smoking and reduce intake of salt and fatty foods.
- Drugs used to treat it aim to increase blood flow to the heart and to reduce the demand on the heart.
- Stenting of coronary arteries or coronary artery bypass surgery can be performed when disease is severe.

3. Mrs Jones is complaining of pain in her calf muscles when she walks up stairs. Examine the arterial system of her lower limbs . . .

Checklist

- Introduce yourself, obtain consent and expose the patient's lower limbs.
- Inspect the legs and feet (front, back and between toes) for scars, ulcers, pallor, hair loss, skin changes.
- Palpate with the back of your hand to compare any differences in temperature between the two legs.
- Palpate for a pulsatile aorta and each of the peripheral pulses on both sides (femoral, popliteal, tibialis posterior and dorsalis pedis).
- Auscultate the abdominal aorta and femoral arteries for bruits.
- Perform Buerger's test.
- Cover and thank the patient.

SBA answers

2 Anatomy, histology and development of the cardiovascular system

1. B
2. C
3. E
4. E
5. C
6. A
7. B
8. C
9. D

3 Cardiac electrophysiology and arrhythmia

10. D
11. C
12. B
13. B
14. B
15. B
16. C
17. E
18. C
19. D

4 The cardiac cyle and control of cardiac output

20. E
21. E
22. D
23. C
24. E
25. C

5 Haemodynamics and vascular function

26. C
27. D
28. C
29. B
30. B
31. B
32. D

6 Integrated control of the cardiovascular system and cardiovascular reflexes

33. D
34. E
35. B
36. C; carotid sinus, not body, contains baroreceptors
37. A
38. B
39. E
40. A
41. B

7 Atherosclerosis and ischaemic heart disease

42. A
43. A
44. A
45. C
46. B
47. A
48. C

8 Heart failure, myocardial and pericardial disease

49. D
50. B
51. C
52. D
53. E

9 Vascular disease

54. A
55. C
56. E
57. D
58. A
59. B
60. D

10 Basic history and examination of the cardiovascular system

61. A
62. A
63. B
64. C

EMQ answers

1. Structure and function of the heart

1. C
2. A
3. H

2. Cardiac electrophysiology and arrythmia

1. E
2. C
3. F
4. E
5. D

3. Vascular function

1. H
2. C
3. E

4. Vascular function

1. H
2. A
3. E

5. Heart failure, myocardial and pericardial disease (this is not specific to Chapter 8)

1. B
2. H
3. C

6. History and examination

1. K
2. J
3. F

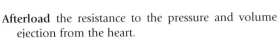

Glossary

Afterload the resistance to the pressure and volume ejection from the heart.

Asystole absence of contraction. Asystole is when the heart has stopped beating and is different from ventricular fibrillation where the heart is still contracting, but not in a coordinated manner.

Bradycardia a heart rate <60 bpm.

Cardiac output (CO) the amount of blood pumped out by the heart every minute, calculated as stroke volume (SV) × heart rate (HR).

Central venous pressure (CVP) the pressure of blood in the great veins as they enter the right atrium.

Contractility the strength with which the myocardium contracts for a given fibre length.

Diastole part of the cardiac cycle where the ventricles are relaxed and filling.

Ectopic an event occurring at a place other than its normal location, for example ventricular ectopics originate from the ventricles, not the sinoatrial node.

End-diastolic pressure (EDP) the pressure in the ventricle at the end of diastole.

End-diastolic volume (EDV) the amount of blood in the ventricle at the end of diastole; the greatest amount found in the ventricle throughout the whole cardiac cycle.

Ejection fraction the proportion of EDV which is ejected by contraction.

Infarction tissue death caused by inadequate perfusion.

Laplace relationship a relationship between the tension, pressure and diameter of a container (implied blood vessel), as tension = diameter × pressure.

Mean arterial pressure (MAP) the average pressure in the system at any point in time, approximated as the diastolic pressure + (1/3 × pulse pressure).

Ohm's law a relationship between resistance, pressure and flow inside a container (implied blood vessel), as pressure = flow × resistance.

Perfusion movement of blood through an organ or tissue.

Preload the degree of ventricular myocyte stretch before contraction. It is determined by the end-diastolic volume.

Sinus rhythm a rhythm under direct control from the sinoatrial node.

Sphygmomanometer a device used for measuring blood pressure.

Starling's law a phenomenon whereby the heart increases its output by increasing its strength of contraction when the fibres of the myocardium are stretched.

Stroke volume (SV) the amount of blood ejected from the left ventricle with each beat.

Stroke work (SW) the amount of external energy expended in one ventricular contraction. SW is the arterial pressure (AP) multiplied by the SV.

Syncope temporary loss of consciousness from reduced blood flow to the brain.

Systemic vascular resistance (SVR) the resistance to blood flow offered by all of the systemic vasculature, excluding the pulmonary vasculature. It is calculated as (MAP–right atrial pressure) / CO.

Systole part of the cardiac cycle where the ventricles are contracting.

Tachycardia a heart rate >100 bpm.

Total peripheral resistance (TPR) the resistance to the flow of blood in the whole system. It is calculated as arterial pressure / cardiac output.

Index

Notes
As the subject of this book is the cardiovascular system, entries under this term have been kept to a minimum: readers are advised to look for more specific terms
vs. indicated a comparison or differential diagnosis
To save space in the index, the following abbreviations have been used:
ECG - electrocardiography/electrocardiogram
Note: Page numbers follwed by *f* indicate figures